Appendicitis - Causes and Treatments

Edited by Elroy Patrick Weledji

Published in London, United Kingdom

Appendicitis - Causes and Treatments
http://dx.doi.org/10.5772/intechopen.1001482
Edited by Elroy Patrick Weledji

Contributors
Elroy Patrick Weledji, George Sakellaris, Xenophon Sinopidis, Konstantinos Zachos, Ioannis Spyridakis, Venkatachalam Raveenthiran, Nagarajan Darun, Shanmugam Shobini, Emmanuel Abiola Babington, Ibrahim Ethem Cakcak, Ahmet Orhan Sunar, Merve Yaren Kayabas, Ndeye Aby Ndoye, Mamadou Mour Traoré, Aloïse Sagna, Aminah Oumou Rassoul Niane, Papa Alassane Mbaye, Florent Tshibwid A. Zeng, Oumar Ndour, Gabriel Ngom, Pratima Gautam, Prakash Mainali, Sandeep Bhattarai, Sunil Kumar Das, Mohamed Mahmoud Eltaweel, Abdulrahman Alotaibi, Vivian E.A. Eta, Nahyeni Bassah, Malika Esembeson, John Ngunde Palle

First published in London, United Kingdom, 2023 by IntechOpen
IntechOpen is the global imprint of INTECHOPEN LIMITED, registered in England and Wales, registration number: 11086078, 5 Princes Gate Court, London, SW7 2QJ, United Kingdom

British Library Cataloguing-in-Publication Data
A catalogue record for this book is available from the British Library

Additional hard and PDF copies can be obtained from orders@intechopen.com

Appendicitis - Causes and Treatments
Edited by Elroy Patrick Weledji
p. cm.
Print ISBN 978-1-83769-747-2
Online ISBN 978-1-83769-748-9
eBook (PDF) ISBN 978-1-83769-746-5

Meet the editor

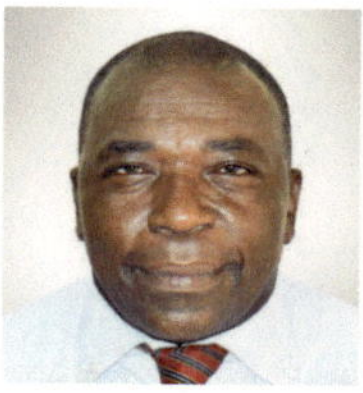

Dr. Elroy Patrick Weledji holds a BSc (Hons) in Physiology, an MSc (Lond) in Neurological Science, an MBBChBAO (Ireland), and an FRCS (Edinburgh). He is currently a Professor of Surgery in the Faculty of Health Sciences at the University of Buea, Cameroon, where his main research interests are gastrointestinal surgery, coloproctology, and surgical oncology. In addition to his academic credentials, Dr. Weledji is a member of the British Association of Surgical Oncology (BASO) and was the first non-European member of the European Society of Coloproctology (ESCP). He has also received fellowships from both organizations, including an ESCP fellowship in pelvic floor surgery in St Gallen, Switzerland, in 2015, and a BASO Ronald Raven fellowship in the Aintree Hepatobiliary Centre in the UK in 2016. Dr. Weledji has published over 150 papers and a book entitled "Theoretical and Clinical Aspects of Surgery in the Tropics". In recognition of his contributions to the field of surgical oncology, he was awarded the Ingeborg Hoerhager Award by the European Federation of Rectal Cancer in 2022.

Contents

Preface **IX**

Section 1
Overview, Causes and Treatment of Appendicitis, and Ultrasound Imaging **1**

Chapter 1 **3**
Appendicitis: Epidemiology, Evaluation, and Controversy in Management
by Elroy Patrick Weledji

Chapter 2 **21**
Acute Appendicitis in Children: Causes and Treatment
by George Sakellaris, Xenophon Sinopidis, Konstantinos Zachos and Ioannis Spyridakis

Chapter 3 **41**
Neglected Appendicitis
by Venkatachalam Raveenthiran, Nagarajan Darun and Shanmugam Shobini

Chapter 4 **71**
Ultrasound Imaging of Appendicitis
by Emmanuel Abiola Babington

Section 2
Management of Complicated Appendicitis and Laparoscopic versus Open Surgery **91**

Chapter 5 **93**
Perforated Appendicitis
by Ibrahim Ethem Cakcak, Ahmet Orhan Sunar and Merve Yaren Kayabas

Chapter 6 **103**
Pediatric Complicated Appendicitis
by Ndeye Aby Ndoye, Mamadou Mour Traoré, Aloïse Sagna, Aminah Oumou Rassoul Niane, Papa Alassane Mbaye, Florent Tshibwid A. Zeng, Oumar Ndour and Gabriel Ngom

Chapter 7 **111**
Treatment of Complicated Appendicitis
by Pratima Gautam, Prakash Mainali, Sandeep Bhattarai and Sunil Kumar Das

Chapter 8 **123**
Laparoscopic versus Open Surgery for Suspected Appendicitis
by Mohamed Mahmoud Eltaweel

Section 3
Current Treatments and Nursing Management of Appendicitis **135**

Chapter 9 **137**
Current Treatments for Appendicitis
by Abdulrahman Alotaibi

Chapter 10 **151**
Nursing Management of Patients with Appendicitis
by Vivian E.A. Eta, Nahyeni Bassah, Malika Esembeson and John Ngunde Palle

Preface

Acute appendicitis, a condition with a lifetime risk of 7%, is the most common surgical emergency. It stands as one of the few conditions that can be treated solely based on clinical findings. *Appendicitis - Causes and Treatments* is a compilation of works by experts in the field of appendicitis and its management. It is divided into three sections, each containing insightful and informative content.

The first section provides a natural history of appendicitis, with Chapter 1 offering an introduction to appendicitis, its epidemiology, evaluation, and the controversies in its management. It emphasizes the difficulty in accurately diagnosing appendicitis and examines the indications and rationale for operative, non-operative (antibiotic) treatment, or both. Furthermore, it delves into the controversy surrounding the management of appendix mass/abscess and the debate between expedient appendicectomy and conservative treatment (antibiotics) with interval appendicectomy.

Chapter 2 discusses the frequency and diagnostic features of complicated appendicitis in children, and explores the various factors that can predict the type of complications that may occur. Chapter 3 examines the theoretical basis of the etiology of acute appendicitis in children. Although laparoscopy has enhanced operative options, non-operative treatments also exist for non-complicated appendicitis.

Chapter 4 demonstrates that ultrasound imaging of appendicitis is operator-dependent. A highly skilled experienced operator using high-quality equipment can diagnose appendicitis with comparable sensitivity and specificity to CT and MRI scanning. In fact, a CT scan is not as effective as ultrasound imaging in diagnosing early appendicitis.

The second section of the book covers the operative and non-operative management of appendicitis and the advantages and disadvantages of the laparoscopic and open approaches to appendicectomy.

The third section summarizes the current treatments for acute appendicitis and the role of nursing care in the perioperative management of patients with appendicitis.

In conclusion, *Appendicitis - Causes and Treatments* is an excellent source of information for anyone seeking to understand the complexities of appendicitis and its management. Enjoy reading!

Elroy Patrick Weledji
Professor of Surgery,
University of Buea,
Buea, Cameroon

Section 1

Overview, Causes and Treatment of Appendicitis, and Ultrasound Imaging

Chapter 1

Appendicitis: Epidemiology, Evaluation, and Controversy in Management

Elroy Patrick Weledji

Abstract

Appendicitis is the most common acute general surgical emergency. As no investigation is accurate, the diagnosis has to rely on clinical symptoms and signs or clinical scoring systems and as a result, frequently misdiagnosed. Blockage of the appendiceal lumen by faecolith is assumed to be the mechanism in many cases. Surgery for appendicitis only evolved when the mortality associated with perforated appendicitis was high. The fact that only few patients progressed to potentially lethal complications provided the argument for conservative antibiotic treatment. The indications for operative (surgery), non-operative (antibiotics), or both in management are discussed. Laparoscopic appendicectomy has become the gold standard of treatment but non-operative management with antibiotics may suffice in selected cases with uncomplicated appendicitis. The controversy in the management of the appendix mass/abscess between an expedient appendicectomy, or a combination of conservative management and interval appendicectomy is discussed. The novel minimally invasive techniques including natural orifice transluminal endoscopic surgery (NOTES) are evolving but for the limitations, cost, availability, and technical expertise required.

Keywords: appendicitis, etiology, assessment, management

1. Introduction

Appendicitis is the most common intra-abdominal emergency. The presentation of acute appendicitis is varied, ranging from subclinical and self-resolving to overwhelming sepsis and death. Typically, patients who develop appendicitis in isolated settings (e.g., on ships, submarines, saturation dives, or in remote areas) are treated conservatively with antibiotics, and, in most cases, appendicitis is resolved without surgery [1–6]. Surgery for the acute abdomen caused by appendicitis only evolved when the mortality associated with perforated appendicitis was found to be significant (>5%). The mortality was associated with the age of the patient and delayed diagnosis resulting in perforated appendicitis [1]. Conservative treatment with later drainage of any abscess had been the standard and diffuse peritonitis was usually fatal. The fact that only few patients progressed to potentially lethal complications provided the argument for conservative antibiotic treatment. Although it is clearly advantageous to spare patients from unnecessary surgery, the morbidity and mortality from failing to diagnose appendicitis until perforation has occurred are greater than that associated with the removal of a normal appendix [2–4]. Thus, early surgery for all patients with suspected appendicitis became the definitive method of preventing severe peritoneal sepsis. However, recent studies particularly during the coronavirus-19 (COVID-19) lockdown have re-iterated the fact that although there is a 20% risk of recurrent attacks, simple appendicitis may be treated with antibiotics only [3, 5]. This may explain the decreased incidence of acute appendicitis during the COVID-19 pandemic following antibiotic treatment for right iliac fossa pain, but the high incidence of complicated appendicitis due to the "stay at home" message [5]. Advances in interventional radiological techniques for peritonitis have also significantly reduced the morbidity and mortality of physiologically severe complicated abdominal infections including appendix abscesses [7].

2. Prevalence

Appendicitis is a global disease. The incidence of appendicitis is 7–12% in the population of the USA and Europe, and, stable in most western countries [8]. Data from newly industrialized countries are sparse but suggest appendicitis is rising rapidly, although it is still lower than the reported incidence amongst patients in the developed world [8–10]. Appendicitis trends in South Africa are consistent with those in developing regions [9]. The lifetime risk of developing acute appendicitis requiring surgery is ~7% which is maximal in childhood and declines steadily with increasing age as the lymphoid tissue and vascularity atrophy [1, 2, 8]. Acute appendicitis can occur at any age but it is rare in infants because of their larger appendiceal ostium. The incidence rises rapidly in children above the age of 5 years and reaches a peak in teenagehood with a median age of 10–11 years [2, 11]. The disease is not uncommon in the elderly and can occur in extreme old age. Some authors have reported a sex difference in the younger age group (15–25 years) where it may be twice as common amongst males. However, it is not surprising that women continue to have a higher appendicectomy rate with 30% revealing normal appendices because of various gynecological conditions mimicking appendicitis [12, 13]. There is still considerable discussion about the reasons why the appendix should so commonly become infected. The fact that its lumen is open to feces and pathogenic organisms of the colon must play an important role, but the main factor that has been implicated is blockage of the lumen by faecolith, by hypertrophy of lymphoid follicles, or by fibrous stricture. This is made more likely by its narrow lumen. Abnormalities of its shape or position (such as occurs, for example, when a short appendicular artery holds the organ up retro-ileally may predispose to infection because of kinking causing obstruction [2]. As long as 1896, it was reported that "iliac phlegmons" were less common in the southern states of America than in the north, and the blacks in northern states had a lower incidence of the disease than whites. This did not appear to be due to genetic factors because when American blacks began moving to the north of the USA in large numbers an increasing incidence of appendicitis occurred. Diet appears to be an important factor in the etiology of infection. In Western countries, 16% of the population undergoes appendicectomy but in Africa and Asia with a high roughage diet, the prevalence is much lower [14]. Burkitt described an increase in disease in Africa associated with the adoption of a Western diet [14]. Walker et al. reported the prevalence of appendicitis in South African students from different racial backgrounds and ascribed the higher incidence to a lower intake of dietary fiber. They also found a marked difference in different social groups. In one study, they reported an annual rate of appendicitis of 7.8 cases per 1000 population of privileged white students eating a typical Western diet, but only 1.8 cases per 1000 in an underprivileged group of white students on a high-fiber diet [15]. The fact that increasing the dietary fiber in modern Western society can reduce the incidence of appendicitis, is demonstrated by the substantial fall over the last 30 years in Western countries. The prevalence has been more or less stable since the year 2000, at 151 per 100,000 person years within Western Europe and assumed to be secondary to improved living standards and general hygiene [8]. Most deaths occur in the elderly because of rapid progression to gangrene, delayed diagnosis, and peritoneal sepsis compounding coincidental cardiovascular, respiratory, or renal pathology [1, 2, 16].

3. Anatomy and pathology

The appendix is a blind-ending hollow muscular tube that arises as a diverticulum from the cecum at the confluence of the taeniae coli. It is thus the beginning of the colon and the structure of its wall comprising serosal, muscular, submucosal, and mucosal layers is not different from the cecum. However, the lumen of the appendix is irregular and narrow due to abundant lymphoid follicles, interspersed with a few mucus-secreting glands in the submucosa. The lymphatic channels in the submucosa tend to run in a longitudinal direction. There is a profuse blood supply via one or two appendicular arteries arising from the ileocolic artery. The arteries run in the mesoappendix, but they are closely applied to the wall distally, and secondary thrombosis is common. The lymphoid tissue and vascularity atrophy with age. In 15–20% of individuals, the appendix is extraperitoneal in a retrocecal position in 64% requiring a retrograde approach in resection. In 80–85%, the position is variable, depending on the length and mobility of the appendix and cecum (preileal 1%, postileal 0.5%, subcecal 2%, and pelvic 32%) although may show variations with different populations [17, 18]. In pregnancy, the enlarging uterus progressively displaces the appendix up into the right hypochondrium [17]. The organ probably has a little function but some authors have suggested that the numerous follicles may indicate that it has important immunological activity in the gut, at least during the first three decades of life when the lymphoid tissue is such a prominent future. This may also suggest a biological cause to the association of appendicectomy with an increased risk of Crohn's disease and, the appendix protecting against ulcerative colitis [19, 20]. Although blockage of the appendiceal lumen is assumed to be the mechanism in many cases of appendicitis, the underlying causative pathology is not always clear, and frequently misunderstood [21]. Inflammation of the appendix is initiated by obstruction of the lumen secondary to swelling of the lymphoid tissue in the wall in response to viral infection or to mechanical obstruction by a faecolith (from a low-fiber diet) in the lumen. Extrinsic compression, inflamed, obstructed, or perforated appendix can occur in a hernia (Amyand's hernia) and previous inflammation may result in fibrotic stricture of the wall. Occasionally, the obstruction may result in a mucocele [22, 23]. Tumors usually present as acute appendicitis or as a mucocele of the appendix caused by obstruction. Less commonly the tumor may present as an abdominal mass causing pain or obstruction. Neoplasms of the appendix and adjacent cecum also cause obstructive appendicitis. Benign neoplasms (leiomyoma, fibroma, neuroma, neurofibroma, and ganglioneuroma) have been recorded but the most common tumor is the carcinoid which occurs in 1% of appendicectomies. Other malignant tumors are uncommon but adenocarcinomas, malignant mucocele, and a variety of sarcoma have been described. A blockage has been observed by parasitic worms and the enlargement of lymphoid aggregates within the appendix wall in Burkitt's (Non-Hodgkin's) lymphoma [24, 25]. Being an extranodal lymphoid organ, it could be the only initial indication of lymphoma or an underlying pathology and, an important reason for routine histological examination of a resected appendix [26]. Acute appendicitis is the commonest indication for surgery in HIV/AIDS and the opportunistic cytomegalovirus (CMV) has been isolated from appendix specimens in these patients raising the possibility that CMV may be causative or a co-factor [27–29]. It may also be due to the obstructing lymphadenopathy from the atypical mycobacterium avium intracellular (MAI) or lymphoma or the immune reconstitution syndrome with the highly active antiretroviral treatment (HAART). These are associated with a high level of immunosuppression and operative mortality. Thus, the importance of liaison with the HIV/AIDS physician in management [30, 31]. The pathology of acute appendicitis is classically described as suppurative, gangrenous, or perforated. The acute inflammation of the appendix ranges from trivial catarrhal inflammation with a complete spontaneous resolution by host defenses, to fatal suppurative necrosis with perforation, abscess formation, or generalized peritonitis. The appendicular artery is a single-end artery closely applied to the wall distally, and secondary thrombosis is common giving rise to gangrene which explains the short progressive history (3–5 days) and the poorer prognosis with the atherosclerosis of the aged. Typically, there is a full-thickness inflammation of the appendix wall, and as the disease progresses hemorrhagic ulceration and necrosis of the wall indicate gangrenous appendicitis and subsequent perforation may be associated with localized peri-appendiceal abscess or generalized peritonitis. The bacteria flora of the appendix comprises the anaerobic and aerobic organisms typical of the large bowel. Luminal obstruction and stercoral ulceration, due to a large faecolith, promote invasive infection, and inflammatory endarteritis. Faecoliths are present in 30–40% of resected appendices, and gangrene is twice as common (75–80%) in these appendices compared to those containing no faecolith [23]. Stump appendicitis is a rare delayed complication of appendicectomy with time intervals ranging from 2 months to 51 years and, is under-reported in the literature [32, 33].

4. Natural history

If appendicitis is untreated, progression of the disease depends on the interplay of several factors (**Table 1**). Progression from intramural inflammation through

Systemic	Local
Extremes of age Coincidental systemic disease (e.g., rheumatoid arthritis, morbid obesity) Immunosuppression (*e.g., as a result of HIV/AIDS, corticosteroids, chemotherapy*)	Site of appendix Speed of development of inflammation Presence of faecolith Vascular impairment Mobility of omentum (less in children)

Table 1.
Factors determining progression of inflammation in appendicitis.

luminal obstruction to gangrene and perforation is not inevitable. Inflammation follows a variable pattern that may be aborted or delayed by host defenses at any time [34]. Children less than 3 years of age have an 80% perforation rate because of delay in diagnosis and host defenses including the omentum are not fully developed [11, 35]. Appendicitis has a more rapid course in the elderly because atherosclerosis, gangrene, and perforation are common [36]. The perforation rate of 25% in patients with a history of pain of less than 24 hours is not much lower than 35% rate of perforation in patients with a history of over 48 hours [37]. An alternative outcome is that the appendix becomes surrounded by a mass of omentum which walls the inflammatory process and prevents inflammation from spreading to the abdominal cavity (appendix mass) yet resolution of the condition is delayed. If the appendix becomes walled off by omentum but has perforated, an abscess will develop localized to the peri-appendiceal region in the right paracolic gutter or the subcecal area of the pelvis. There is no evidence to indicate the proportion of patients likely to develop diffuse sepsis, because antibiotic treatment alters the pattern of disease by replacing the risks of perforation with the lesser risk associated with surgery [22, 23, 37, 38].

5. Investigations

There are no special investigations to confirm appendicitis. As no test is accurate, the diagnosis has to rely on clinical symptoms and signs. The Alvarado score was designed more than two decades ago as a diagnostic score using the clinical features of acute appendicitis for subsequent clinical management [39]. The appropriateness of its routine clinical use is still unclear (**Table 2**). A recent meta-analysis showed its positive role in "ruling out" appendicitis but not in "ruling in" the diagnosis without surgical assessment and further diagnostic testing. It is inconsistent in children and over-predicts the probability of acute appendicitis in women [40]. Alvarado scoring may be valuable in low-resource or primary care centers where imaging is not an option [38]. The adult appendicitis score (ASS) that stratifies patients into three groups (high, intermediate, and low) and thus selective imaging is reliable and renders a low negative appendicectomy rate [41]. It is fast and accurate in categorizing patients with suspected appendicitis, takes into account gender, duration of symptoms, and age, and roughly halves the need for diagnostic imaging (**Table 3**). A right iliac fossa pain treatment (RIFT) study

Symptoms	Migration	1
	Anorexia-acetone	1
	Nausea-vomiting	1
Signs	Tenderness in right lower quadrant	2
	Rebound pain	1
	Elevation of temperature	1
Laboratory	Leukocytosis	2
	Shift to the left	1
Total Score		10

A score of 5 or 6 = acute appendicitis; 7–8 = probable appendicitis; 9–10 = very probable appendicitis.

Table 2.
Alvarado scoring system.

Symptoms and findings		Score
Pain in RLQ	Mild	2
Pain relocation	Moderate or severe	2
RLQ tenderness		3/1*
Guarding		2
		4
Laboratory tests	≥7.2 and <10.9	1
Blood leukocyte count (×10⁹)	>10.9 and <14.0	2
Proportion of neutrophils	≥14.0	3
CRP (mg/l), symptoms <24 h	≥62 and <75	2
CRP (mg/l), symptoms >24 h	≥75 and <83	3
	≥83	4
	≥4 and <11	2
	≥11 and <25	3
	≥25 and <83	5
	≥83	1
	≥12 and <53	2
	≥53 and <152	2
	≥152	1

Table 3.
Adult Appendicitis Score.

group observational study on behalf of the West Midlands Research Collaborative [42] demonstrated that in clinical practice the adult appendicitis score (AAS) can be used more reliably than the Alvarado and the Raja Isteri Pengiran Anak Saleha appendicitis (RIPAS) scoring systems. The Appendicitis Inflammatory Response (AIR) scoring system showed a direct relationship with the phase of acute appendicitis in immigrant patients, but the introduction of the adult appendicitis score (AAS) reduced the negative appendicectomy rate [43, 44]. Tests should serve as adjuncts to clinical diagnosis and may help exclude alternative diagnoses, especially in female or the elderly. A white cell count is usually elevated but a normal white cell count does not exclude appendicitis [39–41]. The appendicolith, a radio-opaque concretion located within the appendix, which is deemed to be the most specific finding of appendicitis on plain radiographs is visualized in only 5–15% of patients with appendicitis [45]. Ultrasonography (US) in expert hands is perhaps the most useful investigation. It has a high specificity (94%), high predictive value, noninvasive, and identifies alternative pathology but of low sensitivity (88%) in early appendicitis [46]. Although computed tomography (CT) scan is superior to US scan and allows for alternative causes of abdominal pain to be diagnosed, the risk of radiation-induced malignancy (21/100,000 patients) renders it not of particular use in pediatric patients. It is expensive and has a low sensitivity (72%) in early and perforated appendicitis [47, 48]. An appendix "triple test" (a combination of negative diagnostic imaging a normal white cell count and normal C-reactive protein can improve diagnostic accuracy significantly without an unacceptable rise in the rates of perforation/gangrenous appendicitis [49, 50]. Laparoscopy is essentially an operation rather than an investigation. Although, usually restricted to young women with equivocal signs many studies have now demonstrated that laparoscopy significantly improves surgical decision-making in patients with acute abdominal pain [12, 13, 36, 38]. The continuing development of ultrasound techniques and laparoscopic surgery have demonstrated that the proportion of normal appendices removed (20%) is unacceptably high [13].

6. Controversy in management

It is not possible to practice fully the ideal management of early diagnosis and surgery for the acute abdomen, thus reducing morbidity and mortality to zero because patients and the disease are variable [16, 51]. Because infection, inadequate perfusion, and a persistent inflammatory state are the most important factors for the development of multiple organ failure it seems logical that initial therapeutic efforts should be directed at their early treatment or prevention (early goal-directed therapy) with intravenous fluids, antibiotics, and analgesia [52, 53]. The risk of portal pyemia from septic emboli is also decreased. It is important to recognize the features of the acute abdomen which would indicate the need for resuscitation in the high dependency or intensive care unit [49, 54].

6.1 Operative or non-operative or both?

Since the incidental removal of an inflamed appendix through a groin incision for a scrotal hernia by Amyand in 1735 and, the first appendicectomy for appendicitis by the French surgeon Mesteivier in 1759, open appendicectomy through a standard right iliac fossa (modified McBurney's gridiron/Lanz) incision at the earliest possible time after the onset of symptoms is the standard treatment of choice. Diffuse peritonitis, which has been diagnosed preoperatively, should be dealt with by formal laparotomy, to allow thorough peritoneal toilet and lavage [1, 21, 37, 38]. Modern techniques with equal efficacy but with minimal postoperative pain, decrease negative appendicectomy rate, decrease surgical site infection, and early return to normal activities include conventional laparoscopic appendicectomy, a single incision (port) laparoscopic appendicectomy, and transluminal (Natural orifice transluminal endoscopic surgery—NOTES) appendicectomy via a trans gastric, colonic, or vaginal approach [55, 56]. NOTES have the advantage of markedly decreasing surgical site infection, hernias, and postoperative pain [55]. Care should be taken during laparoscopy by insisting upon using disposable ports with a vestibular flange to prevent splash back, and by deflating the abdomen prior to port withdrawal because any aerosol emanating from the port entry wound may harbor HIV or COVID-19 [56]. In addition, the cost and technical expertise required in these novel techniques including the numerous limitations of NOTES should be taken into consideration. Recent guidelines stipulate that appendicectomy should be performed laparoscopically unless this is contraindicated [1, 4]. Although conventional laparoscopic appendicectomy has become the gold standard, these innovations are unlikely to render formal open appendicectomy obsolete [53]. In 2012, in the UK, one-third of patients underwent open appendicectomy [57]. Open appendicectomy provides all the valuable skills of abdominal incision, dissection, resection, and abdominal wall closure required by a trainee surgeon. The skills will be useful following conversion of laparoscopic to open surgery [58]. However, unlike laparoscopic surgery, open procedures typically commit the surgeon to proceed to appendicectomy even if the appendix is macroscopically normal on visualization. Thus, the increased take-up of laparoscopy would hypothetically decrease the negative appendicectomy rate [1, 59, 60]. The results of the surgical treatment of appendicitis have improved dramatically during the past decades because of the introduction of more effective antibiotics against both aerobes and anaerobic organisms if peritonitis develops. Prophylactic use of antibiotics (short course i/v metronidazole) perioperatively halved the incidence of surgical site infection with important clinical and economic consequences [61–63]. A single peri-operative dose of antibiotic is sufficient for low-risk cases, but a therapeutic 3-day course is necessary when peritonitis is present.

The role of antibiotic treatment in early non-perforated appendicitis using broad-spectrum i/v ceftriaxone and i/v metronidazole for anaerobes is well known. There is a reasonable body of evidence to support non-operative treatment of appendicitis predating the COVID-19 pandemic [64–70]. There is evidence of low failure rates and minimal recurrence especially in 5–16 year olds [3, 13]. This has been reinforced by papers from the early stages of the COVID-19 pandemic [71–74] that suggested a reasonable alternative option in the right carefully selected patient but with greater reliance on imaging [71, 72]. However, during the pandemic, there was a higher incidence of complicated appendicitis in patients who underwent appendicectomy when compared to those in the prior year which mostly must have been due to the "stay at home" message [73, 74]. Antibiotics, as definitive therapy may be acting in synergy with the host defense mechanisms and thus be most useful in the acute catarrhal phase of appendicitis which usually spontaneously resolves [2, 3]. It would avoid the complications of open appendicectomy and the generally 10% negative appendicectomy rates. Recent trials have shown that antibiotic treatment is a safe first-line approach in CT-confirmed uncomplicated appendicitis (non-gangrenous nor perforated) [71, 72]. Salminen et al. demonstrated in 257 patients between 16 and 60 years old in Finland that using i/v ertepanem for 3 days followed by 7 days oral levofloxacin and metronidazole 75% required no surgery in 1 year and, there was no progression to complicated disease. The recurrence rate was 27% (1 year), 34% (2 years), 35% (3 years), 37% (4 years), and 39% (5 years) [65]. Thus, even with long-term follow-up, the initial treatment with antibiotics is still a safe alternative approach to appendicectomy. The use of antibiotics can also convert acute appendicitis into a semi-elective procedure and avoid the stress of emergency surgery [75–77]. This was demonstrated in the lock-down period during the COVID-19 pandemic which allowed time to obtain the COVID-19 test result [71–74]. It may also exclude COVID-19 as the cause of the abdominal symptoms which is an important differential diagnosis of appendicitis [73]. A much recent study in Amsterdam showed about half of the average population preferred antibiotics over surgical treatment of uncomplicated appendicitis and were willing to accept a high recurrence risk to avoid surgery initially [78]. This is similarly reproduced in the USA [79]. It is important to note that the effects of widespread antibiotics such as drug resistance and opportunistic infections both in the individual patient and the population at large are poorly considered in the literature [80, 81].

There is controversy in the management of the appendix mass/abscess. Some authors believe that the condition is best managed conservatively as the risk of perforation has passed and the removal of the appendix at this late stage can be difficult. Patients with a mass that does not diminish within a short time should be submitted to full intestinal investigations. In older patients, a diagnosis of carcinoma of the cecum, which has obstructed the appendix, must be considered and excluded by a CT scan or colonoscopy [36]. However, conservative management of an appendix mass risks a 30% recurrence of acute inflammation [2, 37, 38]. Sub-acute obstruction may occur and the appendix mass may be confused with a cecal carcinoma in the elderly, Crohn's disease, ileocecal tuberculosis, or an ovarian tumor. Appendix abscess characterized by swinging pyrexia, tachycardia, undulating mass, and being systemically unwell is best treated by surgical intervention through a standard right iliac fossa incision. Residual necrotic appendix is usually found and resected. Tissues and organs adjacent to the abscess cavity will be friable and should be handled with care.

Thus, for a palpable mass presenting pre-operatively the differentiation of a phlegmonous mass from an abscess is not a practical problem because surgery is the correct management for both. In addition, a mass is often detected only after the patient has been anesthesized and paralyzed. Such a policy renders any debate on interval appendicectomy redundant [1, 37, 38]. The operation which may be an appendicectomy, an ileocecal resection, or a hemicolectomy if indicated during the first admission is expeditious and safe, provided steps are taken to minimize postoperative sepsis. The serious consequences of missing a carcinoma in the elderly patient or other pathological lesions such as Crohn's disease, ileocecal tuberculosis, and schistosomiasis are abolished [37, 38, 82]. The controversies with conservative antibiotherapy and drainage of appendix abscess include the optimal timing of the interval appendicectomy which is usually 6–12 weeks [75–77]. There are reports of recurrent appendicitis and increased neoplasms within that interval. Re-operation is associated with a significant incidence of postoperative complications and most patients are not treated by operation unless they develop further trouble. There is no evidence of benefit of lavage over suction alone for postoperative infective complications [83] and the insertion of a drain in the abscess cavity is controversial. Infact, there is a significantly longer operative time and a higher postoperative complication rate (SSI/intra-abdominal abscess) in the irrigation group than in the suction-only group after laparoscopic appendicectomy for uncomplicated appendicitis [84]. Peritoneal and wound drains are of no use. Delayed or non-closure of the skin is not necessary. Apart from the problem of the drain type (open vs. close), the size of the abscess cavity (small vs. large), and the removal time (early vs. late), abdominal drains may cause more problems than they solve. The adhesions that occur in the healing process of the stump or general peritoneal cavity will attract the peritoneal drain (foreign body), prevent adhesions to vascular structures, and physically damage the small bowel or stump causing an enterocutaneous fistula [85, 86]. Drains can mislead the surgeon as they easily get blocked. They are portals for the entry of exogenous bacteria causing surgical site and wound infection [85]. Large bore drains are useful in sepsis following inadequate peritoneal lavage in generalized peritonitis or residual sepsis but should be placed in the appropriate dependent areas of the abdominal cavity such as the paracolic gutters, pelvis away from the intestine [51]. Postoperative peritoneal sepsis may be diffuse and result in intestinal obstruction or a localized, usually pelvic, abscess requiring protracted convalescence. Both complications are the result of poor surgical technique. Untreated pockets of infected peritoneal fluid and failure to remove faecoliths cause postoperative sepsis. If obstruction and sepsis persist, reoperation is indicated. Leakage from the stump of the appendix is an uncommon but serious complication as it causes high pressure, large output fecal fistula which will require an ileocecal resection or a right hemi-colectomy [87]. Although pelvic abscesses could be drained via the rectum, other well-defined abscesses should be drained percutaneously under radiological or ultrasonic guidance followed by a microbiologically guided therapeutic course of antibiotics for 2 weeks [7, 51]. Ruptured appendicitis has been implicated in causing scarring, which can lead to infertility and/or ectopic pregnancy. Appendicectomy is not associated with future infertility in women from scarring, but with an increased risk of ectopic pregnancy [88]. Although, a nationwide cohort study in Finland in 2021 showed no association between complicated appendicitis on the risk of later in vitro fertilization treatment requirement and ectopic pregnancy [89] the argument or early laparoscopic appendicectomy in childbearing age to diagnose and treat appendicitis or complicated salpingitis is still favored over non-operative management.

6.2 The appendix is normal at operation

The terminal 60 cm of the ileum must be delivered to exclude a Meckel's diverticulum, terminal ileitis, and mesenteric adenitis. If the base of the appendix and cecum are healthy, the appendix is removed when ileitis is present. Biopsy and culture of inflamed nodes aid a diagnosis of *Yersinia* infection. The right ovary and tube must be visualized and the extension of the incision, a head down tilt and adequate retraction may be required. Occasionally, fluid leaking from a perforated peptic ulcer down the right paracolic gutter produces clinical findings resembling those of acute appendicitis. A classical appendicectomy incision would reveal bile-staining free peritoneal fluid and a second upper abdominal incision is usually required. Purulent fluid tracking down the right paracolic gutter may also suggest acute cholecystitis. If the clinical diagnosis is equivocal despite investigations, it is best to begin with a low midline incision which could be extended if there is evidence of a perforated peptic ulcer [37, 38]. Prophylactic appendicectomy during the course of another procedure may be justifiable only in young individuals in whom there is a significant risk of appendicitis, but not appropriate in elderly patients [4, 35].

6.3 Tumor is found in the appendix

This will usually be a carcinoid tumor and appendicectomy is the adequate treatment if the tumor is less than 2 cm in diameter. If larger, right hemicolectomy is necessary. Less commonly a tumor may present as an abdominal mass causing pain or obstruction. Whatever histological variant is found, metastases are rare and the development of a carcinoid syndrome is very uncommon. A mucoid carcinoma confined to the appendix may be indistinguishable from a mucocele, but in either cases rupture must be avoided because of peritoneal dissemination resulting in subsequent myxoma peritonei. Occasionally, a tumor may be found unexpectedly during a laparotomy for some other condition [24, 90].

6.4 Chronic appendicitis or "the grumbling appendix"

Patients with true relapsing or chronic appendicitis are rare (1.5% of all cases of acute appendicitis), and often it is difficult to diagnose as the symptoms may be atypical and short-lived. It is thought to be secondary to partial and transient obstruction of the appendix [91, 92]. Although not considered a surgical emergency, it is often a missed diagnosis with complications such as perforation or abscess formation. In the genuine case of chronic appendicitis, the macroscopic appearance of the appendix is abnormal, and thus the diagnosis is best established by laparoscopy, following which the appendix is removed [92, 93]. Minor frequent episodes of right iliac fossa pain "the grumbling appendix" can be caused by threadworms in the appendix [25] or by some conditions other than the appendix. Chronic pain with evidence of organic disease (weight loss, elevated erythrocyte sedimentation rate (ESR) is usually due to Crohn's disease at any age or cecal carcinoma in the elderly or lymphoma or tuberculosis in endemic areas [82]. Pain without signs or abnormal investigations is likely to be due to irritable bowel syndrome, but small bowel studies are still warranted if pain persists, to exclude more unusual causes. If the patient goes on to complain of recurrent episodes of abdominal pain, anorexia, and general malaise and shows tenderness over the appendix, then it is right to advise a planned (elective) appendicectomy [92, 94].

7. Conclusions

Acute appendicitis is one of a relatively dwindling number of conditions in which a decision to operate may be based solely on clinical findings. Laparoscopic appendicectomy is becoming the gold standard of treatment but non-operative management with antibiotics may suffice in selected cases with uncomplicated appendicitis. The advantages of the innovations in minimally invasive and endoscopic surgery are unlikely to render formal open appendicectomy obsolete. The controversy in the management of the appendix mass/abscess remains.

Funding

The author has no sponsor for this research.

Conflict of interests

None.

Ethical approval

The research did not involve patients directly. Thus there was no need for ethical approval.

Consent

None required.

Author details

Elroy Patrick Weledji
Faculty of Health Sciences, Department of Surgery, University of Buea, Cameroon

*Address all correspondence to: elroypat@yahoo.co.uk

References

[1] Baird DLH, Similli C, Vouniseas SK. Acute appendicitis. British Medical Journal. 2017;**357**:1-6

[2] Norman CJ. The pathology of acute appendicitis. Annals of Diagnostic Pathology. 2000;**4**(1):46-58

[3] Flum DR. Clinical practice. Acute appendicitis—appendectomy or the "antibiotics first" strategy. The New England Journal of Medicine. 2015;**372**(20):1937-1943

[4] Di Saverio S. Diagnosis and treatment of acute appendicitis: 2020 update of the WSES Jerusalem guidelines. World Journal of Emergency Surgery: WJES. 2020;**15**(1):27

[5] Tankel J, Keinan A, Blich O, Koussa M, Helou B, Shay S, et al. The decreasing incidence of acute appendicitis during COVID-19: A retrospective multi-centre study. World Journal of Surgery. 2020, Aug;**44**(8):2458-2463

[6] Livingston E, Vons C. Treating appendicitis without surgery. JAMA. 2015;**313**(23):2327-2328

[7] Akinci D, Akhan O, Ozmen MN, Karabulut N, Ozkan O, Cil BE, et al. Percutaneous drainage of 300 intraperitoneal abscesses with long term follow-up. Cardiovascular and Interventional Radiology. 2005;**28**: 744-750

[8] Ferris M, Quan S, Kaplan BS. The global incidence of appendicitis: A systematic review of population-based studies. Annals of Surgery. 2017;**266**(2): 237-224

[9] Yang E, kahn D, Cook C. Acute appendicitis in South Africa: A systematic review. South African Journal of Surgery. 2015;**53**(3740): 31-38

[10] Kong VY, Sartorius B, Clarke DC. Acute appendicitis in the developing world is a morbid disease. Annals of the Royal College of Surgeons of England. 2015;**97**(5):390-395

[11] Huang L, Yin Y, Yang L, Wang C, Li Y, Zhou Z. Comparison of antibiotic therapy and appendectomy for acute uncomplicated appendicitis in children. JAMA Pediatrics. 2017;**171**(5):426-434

[12] Pearse JM. Pelvic inflammatory disease. British Medical Journal. 1990;**300**:1000-1091

[13] Paterson-Brown S, Eckersley JRT. Laparoscopy as an adjunct in decision-making in the acute abdomen. The British Journal of Surgery. 1986;**73**: 1022-1024

[14] Burkitt DP. The aetiology of appendicitis. The British Journal of Surgery. 1971;**58**:675

[15] Walker ARP, Walker BF, Richardson BD, Woolford A. Appendicitis, fibre intake and bowel behavior in ethnic groups in south Africa. Postgraduate Medical Journal. 1973;**49**:243

[16] Weledji EP. Is patient factor more important than surgeon-related factor in sepsis prevention in colorectal surgery? International Journal of Surgery Open. 2018;**12**:29-36

[17] Wiley B, Whitaker R, Borley N. Instant Anatomy. 3rd edition. New Jersey, USA: Wiley- Blackwell; 2005

[18] Mwachaka P, El-busaidy H, Sinkeet S, Ogeng'o J. Variations in the position and length of the vermiform appendix in a black Kenyan population. International Scholarly Research Notices Anatomy. 2014;**2014**:871048

[19] Kaplan GG, Pedersen BV, Andersson RE, et al. The risk of developing Crohn's disease after an appendicectomy: A population-based cohort study in Sweden and Denmark. Gut. 2007;**56910**:1387-1392

[20] Andersson RE, Olaiso G, Tysk C, Ekbom AN. Appendicectomy and protection against ulcerative colitis. The New England Journal of Medicine. 2001;**344**:808-814

[21] Petroianu A, Baroso TVV. Pathophysiology of acute appendicitis. JSM Gastroenterology and Hepatology. 2016;**4**(3):1062

[22] Ivashchuk G, Cesmebasi A, Sorenson EP, et al. Amyand's hernia: A review. Medical Science Monitor. 2014;**20**:140-145

[23] Carr NJ. The pathology of acute appendicitis. Annals of Diagnostic Pathology. 2000;**4**(1):46-58

[24] Ruoff C, Hanna L, Zhi W, Shahzad G, Gotlieb V, Saif MW. Cancers of the appendix: Review of the literatures. ISRN Oncology. 2011;**2011**:728579

[25] Chitnis A, Azimi DY, Sabri S, Dehbri A. Enterobius vermicularis: A parasitic cause of appendicular colic. Cureus. 2020;**12**(6):e8525

[26] Weledji EP, Ngowe NM, Abba JS. Burkitt's lymphoma masquerading as appendicitis—two case reports and review of the literature. World Journal of Surgical Oncology. 2014;**12**:187

[27] Weledji EP, Takere MM, Fon P. A case of toxic megacolon and acute appendicitis in HIV/AIDS. Austin Journal of Clinical Case Reports. 2022;**9**(4):1256

[28] Pasticci MB, Corsi S, Spigarelli F, et al. Acute appendicitis due to cytomegalovirus in an apparently immunocompetent patient: A case report. Journal of Medical Case Reports. 2014;**8**:92

[29] Valerdiz-Casasola S, Fardo-Mindan FJ. Cytomegalovirus infection in a patient with the acquired immunodeficiency syndrome. Gastroenterology. 1991;**101**: 247-249

[30] Mahmoud A, Raza SH, Elshaikh E, Mital D, Ahmed MH. Acute Appendicitis in people living with HIV: What does the emergency surgeon needs to know? SAGE Open Medicine. 2021;**9**: 20503120982461

[31] Weledji EP, Nsagha D, Chichom A, Enoworock G. Gastrointestinal surgery and the acquired immune deficiency syndrome. Annals of Medicine and Surgery (London). 2015;**4**(1):36-40

[32] Thomas SE, Denning DA, Cummings MH. Delayed pathology of the appendiceal stump: A case report of stump appendicitis and review. The American Surgeon. 1994;**60**:842-844

[33] Shin LK, Halpern D, Weston SR, Meiner EM, Katz DS. Prospective CT diagnosis of stump appendicitis. AJR. American Journal of Roentgenology. 2005;**184**:S62-S64

[34] Moss JG, Barrie JL, Gunn AA. Delay in surgery for acute appendicitis. Journal of the Royal College of Surgeons of Edinburgh. 1985;**30**:290-293

[35] Brennan GDG. Paediatric appendicitis: Pathophysiology and

appropriate use of diagnosing imaging. Canadian Journal of Emergency Medicine. 2006;**8**(6):425-432

[36] Hardy K, Ackermann C, Hewitt J. The acute abdomen in the older person. Scottish Medical Journal. 2013;**58**:41-45

[37] Krukowski ZH, O'Kelly TJ. Appendicitis. Surgery. 1997;**15**:76-81

[38] Weledji EP. The dilemma of acute appendicitis. In: Garbuzenko D, editor. Actual Problems of Emergency Abdominal Surgery. Rijeka: IntechOpen; 2016. p. 1-8. Available from: https;//www.intechopen.com/chapters/50645. DOI: 10.5772/63097

[39] Alvarado A. A practical score for the early diagnosis of acute appendicitis. Annals of Emergency Medicine. 1986;**5**(5):557-564

[40] Ohle R, O'Reilly F, O'Brien KK, Fahey T, Dimitrov BD. The Alvarado score for predicting acute appendicitis: A systematic review. BMC Medicine. 2011;**9**:139

[41] Sammalkorpi HE, Mentula P, Savolainen H, leppaniemi A. The introduction of adult appendicitis score reduced negative appendectomy rate. Scandinavian Journal of Surgery. 2017;**106**(3):196-201

[42] RIFT Study Group On behalf of the West Midlands Research Collaborative. Right Iliac fossa Pain Treatment (RIFT) study: Protocol for an international, multicentre, prospective observational study. BMJ Open. 2018;**8**:e017574

[43] Nanjundaiah N, Asfaque M, Venkatesh S, Kaplana A, Priya SA. A comparative study of RIPAS score and ALVARADO score in the diagnosis of acute appendicitis. Journal of Clinical and Diagnostic Research. 2014;**8**(11):NC03-NC05

[44] Von-Muhlen B, Franzon O, beduschi MG, Kruel N, Lupselo D. Appendicitis inflammatory response (AIR) score assessment for acute appendicitis. Arquivos Brasileiros de Cirurgia Digestiva. 2015;**28**(3):171-173

[45] Thorpe JA. The plain abdominal radiograph in acute appendicitis. Annals of the Royal College of Surgeons of England. 1979;**61**(1):45-47

[46] Hussain S, Rahman A, Abassi T, Aziz T. Diagnostic accuracy of ultrasonography in acute appendicitis. Journal of Ayub Medical College, Abbottabad. 2014;**26**(1):12-17

[47] Rogers W, Hoffman J, Noori N. Harms of CT scanning prior to surgery for suspected appendicitis. BMJ Evidence-Based Medicine. 2015;**20**:3-4

[48] Rud B, Vejborg TS, Rappeport ED, Reitsma JB, Wille-Jorgensen P. How accurate is computed tomography for the diagnosis of acute appendicitis in adults? Cochrane Database of Systematic Reviews. 2019;**11**:CD009977

[49] March B, Gillies D, Gair J. Appendicectomies performed > 48 hrs after admission to a dedicated acute general surgical unit. Annals of the Royal College of Surgeons of England. 2014;**96**(8):604-607

[50] Khan MN, Davie E, Inshad K. The role of white cell count and C-reactive protein in the diagnosis of acute appendicitis. Journal of Ayub Medical College, Abbottabad. 2004;**16**(3):17-19

[51] Marik PE. Surviving sepsis: Going beyond the guidelines. Annals of Intensive Care. 2011;**1**(1):17

[52] Weledji EP, Ngowe NM. The challenge of intraabdominal sepsis. International Journal of Surgery (London). 2013;**1194**:290-295

[53] Ruffolo C, Fiorot A, Pagura G, Antonuitti M, Massani M, et al. Acute appendicitis: What is the gold standard of treatment? World Journal of Gastroenterology. 2013;**19**(47): 8799-8807

[54] Nguyen NT, Zainabadi K, Mavandadi S, Paya M, Stevens CM, Root J, et al. Trends in utilization and outcomes of laparoscopic versus open appendectomy. American Journal of Surgery. 2004;**188**:813-820

[55] Bernhardt J, Steffen H, Schneider-Koriath S, Ludwig K. Clinical notes appendectomy study: Comparison of transvaginal notes appendectomy in hybrid technique with laparoscopic appendectomy. International Journal of Colorectal Disease. 2015;**30**(2):259-267

[56] Hanbali N, Herrod PJ, Patterson J. A safe method to evacuate pneumoperitoneum during laparoscopic surgery in suspected COVID-19 patients. Annals of the Royal College of Surgeons of England. 2020;**102**:392-393

[57] National Surgical Research Collaborative. Multicentre observational study of performance variation in provision and outcome of emergency appendicectomy. British Journal of Surgery. 2013;**100**:1240-1252

[58] McBurney C IV. The incision made in the abdominal wall in cases of appendicitis, with a description of a new method of operating. Annals of Surgery. 1894;**20**(1):38-43

[59] Foster GE, Burke JB, Bolwell J, Doran J, Balfour TW, Holliday A, et al. Clinical and economic consequences of wound sepsis after appendicectomy and their modification by metronidazole or povidone iodine. Lancet. 1981;**1**:769

[60] Eriksson S, Granstrom L. Randomized controlled trial of appendicectomy versus antibiotic therapy for acute appendicitis. The British Journal of Surgery. 1995;**82**:166-169

[61] Styrud J, Eriksson S, Nilsson I. Appendectomy versus antibiotic treatment in acute appendicitis. A prospective multicenter randomized controlled trial. World Journal of Surgery. 2006;**30**:1033-1037

[62] Hansson J, Korner U, Khorram-Manesh A, Solberg A, Lundholm K. Randomized clinical trial of antibiotic therapy versus appendicectomy as primary treatment of acute appendicitis in unselected patients. The British Journal of Surgery. 2009;**96**:473-481

[63] Turhan AN, Kapan S, Kutukcu E, Yigitbas H, Hatipoglu S, Aygun E. Comparison of operative and non-operative management of acute appendicitis. Ulus Travma Acil Cerrahi Derg [The Turkish Journal of Trauma and Emergency Surgery]. 2009;**15**: 459-462

[64] Vons C, Barry C, Maitre S. Amoxicillin plus clavulanic acid versus appendicectomy for treatment of acute uncomplicated appendicitis: An open-label, non-inferiority, randomised controlled trial. Lancet. 2011;**377**:1573-1579

[65] Salminen P, Paajanen H, Rautio T. Antibiotic therapy vs appendectomy for treatment of uncomplicated acute appendicitis: The APPAC randomized

clinical trial. Journal of the American Medical Association. 2015;**313**:2340-2348

[66] Park HC, Kim MJ, Lee BH. Randomized clinical trial of antibiotic therapy for uncomplicated appendicitis. The British Journal of Surgery. 2016;**104**:1785-1790

[67] Neufeld MY, Bauerle W, Eriksson E. Where did the patients go? Changes in acute appendicitis presentation and severity of illness during the coronavirus disease 2019 pandemic: A retrospective cohort study. Surgery. 2021;**169**(4): 808-815

[68] Mason RJ, Moazzez A, Sohn H, Katkhouda N. Meta-analysis of randomized trials comparing antibiotic therapy with appendectomy for acute uncomplicated (no abscess or phlegmon) appendicitis. Surgical Infections. 2012;**13**:74-84

[69] Varadhan KK, Neal KR, Lobo DN. Safety and efficacy of antibiotics compared with appendicectomy for treatment of uncomplicated acute appendicitis: Meta-analysis of randomised controlled trials. BMJ. 2012;**244**:e2156

[70] Findlay JM, el Kafsi J, Hammer C, Gilmour J, Gillies RS, Maynard ND. Non-operative management of appendicitis in adults: A systematic review and meta-analysis of randomized controlled trials. Journal of the American College of Surgeons. 2016;**223**:814-824.e2

[71] Javanmard-Emamghissi H, Boyd-Carson H, Hollyman M. The management of adult appendicitis during the COVID-19 pandemic: An interim analysis of a UK cohort study. Techniques in Coloproctology. 2021;**25**:401-411

[72] Bowen JM, Jonatheon RC, Sheen RT, et al. Acute appendicitis in the COVID-19 era: A complicated situation? Annals of Medicine and Surgery, (Lond) 2021, 67: 102536

[73] Association of Upper GI Surgery of Great Britain and Ireland (AUGIS). AUGIS Guidelines: Management Algorithm for Patients with Clinically Suspected Appendicitis During Covid-19 Pandemic. London, UK: Association of Surgeons of Great Britain & Ireland; 2020

[74] Association of Surgeons of Great Britain & Ireland Association of Coloproctology of Great Britain & Ireland, Association of Upper Gastrointestinal Surgeons, Royal College of Surgeons of Edinburgh, Royal College of Surgeons of England, Royal College of Physicians and Surgeons of Glasgow, Royal College of Surgeons in Ireland. London, UK: Updated intercollegiate general surgery guidance on COVID-19. 2020. Available from: https://www.rcseng.ac.uk/coronavirus/joint-guidance-for-surgeons-v2/

[75] Kim M, Kim SJ, Cho HJ. Effect of surgical timing and outcomes for appendicitis severity. Annals of Surgical Treatment and Research. 2016;**91**(2):85-89

[76] Ditillo MF, Dziura JD, Rabinovici R. Is it safe to delay appendectomy in adults with acute appendicitis? Annals of Surgery. 2006;**244**:656-660

[77] Jeon BG, Kim HJ, Jung KH, Lim HI, Kim SW, Park JS, et al. Appendectomy: Should it be performed so quickly? The American Surgeon. 2016, Jan;**82**(1):65-74

[78] Bom W et al. Population preference for treatment of uncomplicated appendicitis. Colorectal Disease. 2022;**24**(Supp. 3):22-47

[79] Hanson AL, Crosby RD, Basson MD. Patient preferences for surgery or

antibiotics for the treatment of acute appendicitis. JAMA Surgery 2018, 1;153(5):471.

[80] Elder DP, Kuentz M, Holm R. Antibiotic resistance: The need for a global strategy. Journal of Pharmaceutical Sciences. 2016;**105**(8):2278-2287

[81] Weledji E, Weledji EK, Assob JC, Nsagha DS. Pros, cons and future of antibiotics. New Horizons in Translational Medicine. 2017;**4**(1): 9-14

[82] Weledji EP, Pokam T. Abdominal tuberculosis: Is there a role for surgery? World Journal of Gastrointestinal Surgery. 2017;**9**(8):174-181

[83] Moore CB, Smith RS, Herbertson R, Toeves C. Does use of intraoperative irrigation with open or laparoscopic appendectomy reduce post-operative intra-abdominal abscess? The American Surgeon. 2011;**77**:78-80

[84] Lee TG, Nam S, Lee SH, Lee JH, Homg YK, Kang JG. Irrigation versus suction alone during laparoscopic appendectomy for uncomplicated acute appendicitis. Annals of Coloproctology. 2020;**36**(1):30-34

[85] Rather SA, Shams Bari SUL, Malik AA, Khan A. Drainage vs no drainage in secondary peritonitis with sepsis following complicated appendicitis in adults in the modern era of antibiotics. World Journal of Gastrointestinal Surgery. 2013;**5**(11):300-305

[86] Gusman-Valdivia GG, Linares-Rivera E. Prophylactic drainage in abdominal surgery in adults: True utility? Cirujano General. 2018;**40**(2):105-111

[87] Weledji EP. Perspectives on enterocutaneous fistula: A review article. Medical & Clinical Reviews. 2017;**3**:5

[88] Elraiyah T, Hashim Y, Elamin M, Erwin PJ, Zarroug AE. The effect of appendectomy in future tubal fertility and ectopic pregnancy: A systematic review and meta-analysis. Journal of Surgical Research. 2014;**192**(2):368-374

[89] Mannisto J, Sammalkorpi H, Niinimaki M, Mentula M, Mentula P. Association of complicated appendicitis on the risk of later in vitro fertilization treatment requirement and ectopic pregnancy: A nationwide cohort study. Acta Obstetricia et Gynecologica Scandinavica. 2021;**100**(8):1490-1496

[90] Bucher P, Mathe Z, Demirag A, Morel P. Appendix tumours in the era of laparoscopic appendectomy. Surgical Endoscopy. 2004;**18**(7):1063-1066

[91] Shah S, Gaffney R, Dykes T, Goldstein J. Chronic appendicitis: An often forgotten cause of recurrent abdominal pain. The American Journal of Medicine. 2013;**126**:e7-e8

[92] Mussak T, Scmidbaue S, Nerlich A, Schmidt W, Hallfeldt K. Chronic appendicitis as an independent clinical entity. Chirurg. 2002;**73**:710-715

[93] Kothadia JP, Katz S, Ginzburg L. Chronic appendicitis: Uncommon cause of chronic abdominal pain. Therapeutic Advances in Gastroenterology. 2015;**8**(3):160-162

[94] Royster RL. The grumbling appendix. BMJ; 4 August 1979;**2**(6185):294

Chapter 2

Acute Appendicitis in Children: Causes and Treatment

George Sakellaris, Xenophon Sinopidis, Konstantinos Zachos and Ioannis Spyridakis

Abstract

Acute appendicitis is the most common cause of acute abdomen in children. One-third of patients are under the age of 18 years, with a peak of incidence during puberty. The particular issues of acute appendicitis in childhood are discussed in this chapter. Anatomical variations, such as malrotation, affect clinical presentation during this period. Complicated appendicitis is a rule in children of preschool age. The theoretical basis of etiology of acute appendicitis is discussed as well. While the prevailing theory considered inflammation secondary to obstruction of the appendiceal lumen, during the last two decades, primary infection is gaining ground as the initial trigger of appendicitis. Finally, therapeutic options are discussed, as non-operative treatment is the new issue in non-complicated appendicitis, while operative options have been enhanced with the advent of laparoscopy.

Keywords: acute appendicitis, children, primary infection, causes, treatment

1. Introduction

Acute appendicitis is one of the most common diagnostic and therapeutic issues in pediatric patients. The fact that there are still children with peritonitis, in the era of highly accurate diagnostic modalities, constitutes a challenge for the present generation of clinicians and researchers. The pediatric population is per se a different world, with specific particularities and needs. The scope of the present chapter is to bring to light these particularities, providing incentives for novel ideas against this universal infectious and surgical disease.

2. Embryology, anatomy, and physiology

The appendix forms the last segment of the cecum and begins to differentiate during the 8th week of gestation. During maturation of the primitive intestine, the appendix does not follow the growth of the cecum, which is 4.5 times bigger than the appendix at birth and continues to increase in size until it becomes 8.5 bigger in adults. Throughout the development of the cecum in the gestational life, the appendix along with the anterior colic taenia moves toward the midline of the cecum. In 15% of the population, there is not such a movement, and the appendix presents a funnel shape. Intestinal villi can be observed between the 4th and 5th month of gestation but vanish before birth. At the 7th month of fetal life, lymphatic nodules appear. They increase in number until puberty, and then a decline is noticed. After the 60th year of life, there is no lymphatic tissue in the appendix in the majority of population, while often the lumen of the appendix vanishes completely [1, 2]. Many claim that the appendix is a vestigial organ without a precise function, while others that it is part of the GALT (Gut-Associated Lymphoid Tissue) system, containing M cells, which can produce IgA in response to antigens [3].

The location of the appendix is usually retrocecal (20–74%). Some believe that this happens, because of the rotation of the right colon and cecum around their longitudinal axis [4], while others believe that the appendix is found more often in a retrocecal position as a result of its formation and shaping during the descent of the cecum [5]. There are also the pelvic (3.7–58%), pre-ileal (1–50.9%), post-ileal (0.4–14.8%), paracolic (2.9–8%), and retrocolic (1.25–9%) locations [6].

Since the cecum does not possess a true mesentery, initially, it was believed that this was applicable for the appendix too. However, there is a mesoappendix, which contains the appendicular artery. The mesoappendix is a small mesenteric fold, originating from the posterior surface of the mesentery of the distal part of the ileum. Occasionally, the mesoappendix is shorter than the appendix itself, and for that reason, the appendix presents a curve in its longitudinal axis.

The appendicular artery originates from the ileocolic artery, which arises from the colic artery, being usually a solitary one. Nonetheless, it has been reported that appendicular blood supply is multiple, with arteries originating from the anterior and posterior cecal arteries and from the ileocecal artery [2]. From these arteries, collateral blood vessels create, through various anastomoses, a blood network as an alternative blood supply. Such a network is responsible for the multiple variations of the vascularization of the appendix depicted in human anatomy atlases. The appendicular veins run through the mesoappendix and, after merging with the cecal veins, create the ileocolic vein, which drains into the right colic vein. The lymphatic vessels of the appendix through a series of lymph nodes of the appendicular, ileocolic, and superior mesenteric artery drain in the Haller's tripod lymph nodes.

The appendix is innervated by the sympathetic and the parasympathetic systems. The first derives from the superior mesenteric ganglia and from those of Haller's tripod, while the latter originates from the pneumogastric nerve. The knowledge of the different innervation of the visceral and parietal peritoneum is very important to comprehend the distinct kind of pain in case of inflammation in the peritoneal cavity. Initially, inflammation in the right iliac fossa, through the sympathetic innervation of the visceral peritoneum, will create a dull, light pain around the umbilicus. Once the inflammation affects the parietal peritoneum, the characteristic, sharp, continuous pain in the low right abdominal quadrant will emerge, due to sensory nerve fibers, which arise from the 8th thoracic nerve.

3. Congenital malformations

Absence of the appendix is a rarity [7]. An ectopic position of the appendix is a part of congenital malformations affecting the formation of the gastrointestinal tract such as malrotation or situs inversus. A non-fixed cecum with a long mesentery may result in an appendix far away from the right iliac fossa. Surgeons have described lumbar appendicitis, while others found the appendix in the thorax in diaphragmatic hernia [8, 9].

Duplication of the appendix is another uncommon anomaly. The most famous classification of this anomaly is that of Cave and Wallbridge, according to which there can be a partial or total duplication of the appendix with or without the duplication of the cecum and, even, a horseshoe appendix [10]. Diverticula of the appendix have been reported [11]. Ectopic pancreatic, gastric, and esophageal tissues have been found in the appendiceal mucosa [12].

4. Incidence

Acute appendicitis is the most common cause of acute abdomen. In the developed world, 5.7–50 per 100,000 inhabitants are affected by acute appendicitis every year [13]. The incidence of acute appendicitis is declining [14] and presents seasonal variation [15] and significant differences between developed and developing countries. The lifetime risk for acute appendicitis in Europe is 8%, in the USA 9%, and 2% in Africa [16]. One-third of patients with appendicitis are younger than 18 years old, with a peak incidence between the ages of 11 and 12 years [17]. Perforation rates vary from 16% to 40%, occurring more frequently in younger age groups (40–57%) and in patients older than 50 years (55–70%) [18].

It is well known, especially for children, that there may be an atypical presentation of the pain in acute appendicitis, with signs and symptoms, which not only are different from those of the adult population, overlapping with symptoms characteristic for other diseases, and creating a vast catalog of differential diagnosis [19]. This is particularly true for children younger than 5 years old, resulting in erroneous or delayed diagnosis in 5.9–84% of the cases and consequently in complicated appendicitis in 5–51% of the patients. Surprisingly, in children younger than 3 years, the incidence of perforated appendicitis is reported up to 100% [20]. On the other hand, overdiagnosis and consequently unnecessary appendicectomy can reach 23% regarding both child and adult population [21].

5. Etiology and pathophysiology

It is common knowledge that the obstruction of the lumen of the appendix is the main cause of acute appendicitis. However, such an obstruction cannot always be explained [22]. Researchers showed that microbial infection is the main cause of the obstruction of the appendiceal lumen, a fact that explains the presence of acute appendicitis in clusters with seasonal variations and the rare presentation of the disease in rural areas of developing countries [23, 24]. Obstruction can be caused by a foreign body (seed, pin, jewel, etc.), by a carcinoid of the appendix, parasites (*Entamoeba*, *Strongyloides*, *Enterobius vermicularis*, *Schistosoma*, and *Ascaris*), by the increase of the lymphatic tissue due to a bacterial (Yersinia, Salmonella, and Shigella), or a viral infection (enterovirus, cytomegalovirus, measles, varicella, etc.). Moreover, there are reported cases of acute appendicitis following abdominal trauma (the most famous victim was Harry Houdini). Patients with cystic fibrosis have a greater chance of being affected by acute appendicitis as a result of the higher viscosity of the enteric fluids [25].

Obstruction will result in the formation of a "closed" enteric loop and, finally, the perforation of the appendix and the presence of peritonitis. The lumen of a normal appendix can accommodate 0.1 mL of contents, but a volume of 0.5 mL of mucus can raise the intraluminal pressure of the appendix to 60 cm H_2O [26]. The appendix can continue to produce mucus even with an intraluminal pressure of 93 cm H_2O [17]. In such an environment, microorganisms can proliferate rapidly, and as a result, the pressure inside the lumen of the appendix increases even more, compromising initially the function of the lymphatic vessels. The wall of the appendix becomes thicker until there is venous stasis. At a certain point, the arterial blood supply shall decrease, starting from the antimesenteric side of the organ, causing necrosis and, ultimately, perforation.

Histopathological findings have shown scars on the wall of the appendix, indicating older inflammation of the appendix, which did not result in perforation. Thus, some believe that appendicitis can regress without treatment [27].

In order to classify the severity of the inflammation, grading systems have been adopted. One of the most famous is the laparoscopic classification. This grading system correlates the macroscopic appearance with the histopathological examination and the biochemical analysis of the peritoneal fluid. The resulting score includes normal looking appendix (grade 0), hyperemia and edema (grade 1), fibrinous exudate (grade 2), segmental necrosis (grade 3A), base necrosis (grade 3B), abscess (grade 4A), regional peritonitis (grade 4B), and diffuse peritonitis (grade 5) [24]. Grades 1–2 are characterized as non-complicated appendicitis, while grades 3–5 as complicated [28].

The necessary period of time that acute appendicitis evolves to peritonitis due to perforation of the wall depends on various factors such the gender, the age, the body mass index, and concurrent diseases. Although there is no precise rule, theoretically, the rupture of the appendix occurs 24–36 h since the onset of the first symptoms, and the formation of an abscess after 2–3 days [29].

6. Diagnosis

Although acute appendicitis is a well-known pathological entity for centuries, its early diagnosis is still a challenge, especially if the patient is a child. Despite technological innovations and the use of specialized hematological tests and imaging methods, the percentage of prompt diagnosis has not changed during the last decades. Furthermore, children compose a very unique population, since they often cannot provide accurate information nor cooperate adequately [30], resulting in late diagnosis with increased chance of peritonitis.

For this reason, the combination of a detailed history, a thorough physical examination, and appropriate laboratory tests is necessary for a prompt diagnosis. Moreover, repeating the clinical examination and the laboratory analysis, especially performed by the same physician for every single case, is probably the best way to avoid a late or erroneous diagnosis, particularly for the pediatric population for the mentioned reasons.

6.1 Clinical signs and symptoms

Initially, patients with acute appendicitis present mild symptoms for the gastrointestinal system, such as loss of appetite, dyspepsia, and changes of bowel movements. However, the main and first symptom of appendicitis is abdominal pain. Thus, if a severe symptom precedes pain, other pathologies should be taken in consideration [17]. Most studies claim that anorexia occurs at the same time with pain [26]. This is especially true for the pediatric population. Many surgeons concur that a child who is hungry rarely suffers from acute appendicitis.

At first, the pain is localized at the periumbilical area and is described as dull and not very intense. It can be continuous or intermittent. Although it is not a precise rule, after a few hours, due to the irritation of the parietal peritoneum, it migrates to the right iliac fossa and more specifically at the McBurney point, which is found in the proximal third of the imaginary line that connects the anterior superior iliac spine with the umbilicus. Except McBurney point, on the same imaginary line between the anterior superior iliac crest and the umbilicus, two other points have been described as a sign of acute appendicitis, the Morris (Kummel) and the Monro point. Accordingly, in the proximal third of the straight line between the right and left iliac fossa, another pressure point that emits pain is called the Lanz point, while in the same line, but at the right rim of the rectus abdominis muscle, the Clado point.

In addition, the exact position of the appendix can affect not only the location of the abdominal pain, as described, but also its intensity. For example, a retrocecal inflamed appendix can produce pain at a later stage compared with a pre-ileal one, mainly in the right lateral abdominal area and even in the lumbar area.

Certain maneuvers can be used, to trigger pain, which will give suspicion to an inflamed appendix. The pain felt at the right iliac fossa, with the continuous palpation of the left iliac fossa and the migration of the palpation in the direction of the left colic curve, is called the Rovsing sign. The pain sensed in the right abdominal area, after the abrupt cessation of a deep palpation, is known as the Blumberg or rebound sign, not to be confused with the pain felt during the percussion of the same area, called Mandel-Razdolski sign. Both are indicative of peritoneal inflammation. Other signs are the Sitkovskiy (Rosenstein) and Bartomier/Michelson signs. The first is observed when tenderness in the right lower quadrant increases as the patient moves from the supine position to a recumbent posture on the left side. The second regards increased pain during palpation of the right iliac region, as the person being examined lies on their left side compared with the supine position. Obturator sign is defined the discomfort felt by the patient on the slow internal movement of the hip joint while the knee is flexed, because of an inflamed pelvic appendix that contacts the nearby obturator muscle. In case of retrocolic appendicitis overlying the right psoas muscle, the pain elicited by the posterior flexion of the right thigh while lying on the left side is called the psoas sign. Finally, Dunphy and Rotter signs are positive, when pain is felt at the right iliac fossa while the patient is trying to cough and during rectal examination, respectively. The last one means that the inflamed appendix presents probably a direction toward the pelvis.

The position of the appendix is, also, responsible for symptoms that have no relation to the right iliac fossa. For example, dysuria or diarrhea can be present in case of pelvic or retrocolic appendicitis, respectively. A retrocolic inflamed appendix, especially in patients with a non-fixated cecum or a cecum in high position near the liver, can create abscess in the subhepatic area, causing the formation of fluid in the thorax and consequently empyema. Such a condition, although infrequent, is seen mostly in children [31].

It is very important to distinguish between voluntary and involuntary contraction of the abdominal wall, especially in children. The first is a defensive mechanism caused by the fear of the coming palpation while the latter indicates inflammation of the visceral peritoneum.

Patients with acute appendicitis tend to minimize their movements, in order to sooth the pain. During ambulation, they flex the thorax and knees, and they bend laterally toward the right side in order to diminish the pressure of the abdominal muscles and consequently the pain. For the same reason, on the examination table, children may flex their knees to their thorax, assuming a fetal position.

Another important symptom is fever, initially low, and as the inflammation is aggravating, the temperature overcomes 38.5°C. A high temperature since the beginning of symptoms is a sign of an early complicated appendicitis or, more commonly, another disease.

Although vomit is a symptom of all patients with acute appendicitis, it is one of the characteristic symptoms of children, especially of preschoolers, having a neurological etiology, and not caused by obstruction.

Of course, all the symptoms and signs can present in a variety of combinations. The extremely increased probability of complicated appendicitis with high fever, severe vomiting, early intestinal obstruction, and dehydration, in children younger than 3 years, seems to be caused by the low percentage of intraperitoneal fat and the underdeveloped omentum, which cannot confine the expansion of the inflammation and limit the purulent leakage of a ruptured appendix [32].

6.2 Laboratory examinations

The most used blood tests for the diagnosis of acute appendicitis are the count of white blood cells (WBC), the percentage of neutrophils, and the value of the c-reactive protein (CRP), a glycoprotein produce by the liver, as a response to any acute infection. There are many biomarkers used for the diagnosis and even the staging of acute appendicitis in children, among them bilirubin, procalcitonin, calprotectin, aptoglobin, interleukine-8, and serum urokinase-type plasminogen activator receptor [30, 33–35].

All the above hematological biomarkers, taken in consideration alone or in combinations, present a vast range of specificity and sensitivity; however, none of them can diagnose and/or define the severity of the appendicitis with absolute precision. According to modern international guidelines, the various biochemical markers are only a promising predictive tool for the diagnosis of acute appendicitis [36].

These guidelines affirm that children with pain in the right iliac fossa, WBC more than 16,000/mm^3 and CRP more than 10 mg/L, have a high probability for acute uncomplicated appendicitis [36]. Without being a precise rule, greater values of WBC and CRP are indicative of a ruptured appendix. It is important to remember that combined values of WBC, neutrophil count, and CRP within the normal range, are against the possibility of acute appendicitis [37]. To achieve an early and accurate diagnosis, the biomarkers should be taken in consideration always in accordance with the clinical examination and the imaging methods.

6.3 Imaging techniques

The most used imaging methods are simple radiography imaging, ultrasonography, computed tomography (CT), and magnetic resonance imaging (MRI).

Despite the fact that an X-ray is not very important for the diagnosis of the acute appendicitis, it can, however, show indirect evidence of an inflamed appendix, such as a non-structural scoliosis with the curvature toward the right side, in order to alleviate the pain. The absence of the psoas muscle in a simple radiograph is a sign of fluid due to inflammation in the area. Fecal stasis and intestinal obstruction can be easily observed through an X-ray. Radiopaque urinary stones give an easy diagnosis of urolithiasis, while a radiopaque fecalith is very specific in highlighting an obstructed appendiceal lumen. We must not forget that an X-ray of the thorax is crucial in the diagnosis of right-sided pneumonia, which can have as initial symptom the pain in the right abdomen.

Ultrasound is considered the first line imaging method for the diagnosis of acute appendicitis in children. Researchers report a range of specificity and sensitivity of 55–96% and 85–98%, respectively [38, 39]. The fact that this technique is economic, fast, and without radiation makes it the optimal investigation tool for the pediatric population. Ultrasound can measure the length and the diameter of the appendix, detect fluid, stones, fecaliths, air-fluid levels, and abscesses. Besides the appendix, ultrasound can give information about most of the intraperitoneal organs and exclude pathologies that make part of the differential diagnosis of the appendicitis, such as ovarian or epiploic torsion and extrauterine pregnancy. This imaging method has been very helpful in reducing overdiagnosis and consequently unnecessary appendicectomies. However, ultrasound has certain limitations. Firstly, it is an operator-dependent technique, meaning that experience is very important. Secondly, the presence of gas in the intestinal loops and obese patients may reduce its accuracy [40]. Finally, in many medical facilities, the necessary equipment is not always available on a 24-h basis.

FAST (focused assessment with sonography for trauma) is a kind of ultrasound used in trauma. With FAST as a starting point, POCUS (point-of-care ultrasound) was invented. This is a new type of ultrasound that uses a portable device and has already been introduced in the routine examination of many different medical specialties, especially in the emergency departments.

CT is another imaging method for the diagnosis of the acute appendicitis. With this technique, the inspection of the whole intraperitoneal cavity and the retroperitoneal space is possible. It can easily measure not only the diameter, but also the thickness of the appendix, which is considered pathological if greater than 1 mm. It can, also, detect the inflamed fat tissue with more accuracy compared with the ultrasound and can differentiate acute appendicitis from an inflamed Meckel diverticulum. Its accuracy is 90–98% with a specificity of 85–94% and a sensitivity of 92–97%.

To perform a CT, the use of the necessary radiocontrast can create an allergic reaction, and, also, a certain dose of anesthesia is needed, especially for the younger children. However, the main limitation of this imaging method in children is the presence of ionizing radiation. During the international congress for the creation of the guidelines for the diagnosis and treatment of acute appendicitis, there was a strong debate concerning the application of the CT in the pediatric population. Some affirm that the CT with low radiation (2 mSv instead of the normal 4.44 mSv) can be used safely in children with good results in children [41]. It is universally accepted that the use of ionizing radiation for the visualization of the appendix in children must be used a third-line imaging procedure when other routine clinical and laboratory tests are inconclusive [36].

MRI is an excellent diagnostic method for the diagnosis of acute appendicitis due to the absence of any harmful radiation. Studies showed that MRI has analogous specificity and sensitivity as a CT [42]. However, it is more expensive than the ultrasound and the CT. Moreover, it depends a lot on local availability of the equipment and expertise of the personnel. Likewise, the presence of an anesthesiologist is essential for the completion of the diagnostic test. International guidelines suggest the use of MRI as the preferable imaging method for the visualization of the appendix in children, after ultrasound, based on local resources, to avoid the ionizing radiation of a CT [36]. Some also affirm that an appropriate clinical and/or staged algorithm based on US/MRI implementation with a sensitivity up to 98% and a specificity up to 97% can reduce the use of CT [43].

7. Scoring systems

Scoring systems provide an easy instrument for the diagnosis of acute appendicitis. They are predictive tools that take in consideration clinical symptoms, signs, and laboratory test values [44]. In all scoring systems for every feature a specific point is ascribed, in case of positive feedback. The sum will attribute to a specific possibility of acute appendicitis. Each of these predictive tools has a different specificity and sensitivity. The most known scoring systems are the Alvarado score (ALV), Adult Inflammatory Score (AIR), the Adult Appendicitis Score (AAS), the Samuel's Pediatric Appendicitis Score (PAS), and the RIPASA (Raja Isteri Pengiran Anak Saleha Appendicitis) scoring system [45–49]. This last one, initially, was used for the prediction of acute appendicitis in the Asia population. The most used of them in children are the Alvarado and the PAS. PAS is very similar to the Alvarado, although it considers the pain elicited during percussion or coughing more important than leukocytosis. Even though many studies report the importance of these two scoring systems for the diagnosis of acute appendicitis in children, a systematic review of the literature has proven that PAS and ALV over-diagnose the disease by 35% and 32%, respectively. Also, both failed to achieve the predictive performance of the CRP [50]. As mentioned, children in preschool age have atypical symptoms and more complications. In this age group, ALV and PAS present lower scores in comparison with older children [51]. Thus, many have started to use the AIR, which includes fewer symptoms, but takes into consideration the CRP. This scoring system seems to have a better predictive ability for the diagnosis of appendicitis than ALV and PAS [52]. The use of PAS in children demonstrated a specificity of 89% in female adolescents and 78% for the rest of the patients, while the prognostic value was low in both groups [53].

Regarding the severity of the inflammation of the appendix in the pediatric population and the presence of complications, the three features of the ALV with the higher sensitivity, for complicated appendicitis, were the fever, the leukocytosis, and the pain in the right lower quadrant (88.6%, 82.3%, and 79.7% respectively), while the best predictive value for a ruptured appendix was presented by the rebound tenderness [54].

These scoring systems are very helpful, primarily for the exclusion of acute appendicitis, but should not be solely used for the diagnosis of the disease in children [36].

8. Treatment

8.1 Non-operative management

During the last decade, many studies reported that the treatment of acute non-complicated appendicitis is possible without the need of operation in adults and children. Especially for children, only 19% of the patients present a rupture appendix [36, 55]. The success rate for non-operative management with antibiotics was found between 89.2% and 97% of the cases and during a follow-up of 8 weeks up to 4 years, the effectiveness of this conservative treatment was 75.7–79% [56, 57]. Moreover, a systematic review of 2019, which put in comparison appendicectomy to conservative treatment in children with uncomplicated appendicitis, showed that non-operative management (a cure within 2 weeks of intervention) was successful in 58–100% of the cases, with 0.1–31.8% recurrence at 1 year [58], without increasing the risk of complications [59, 60]. With non-operative initial management for simple appendicitis in children, the reported outcomes include less morbidity, fewer disability days, and lower costs when compared with surgery [61].

On the other hand, some argue that conservative management is not as effective as surgery in all pediatric patients with appendicitis, although it seems that such a statement is true if conservative treatment is, also, applied in children with a fecalith in the lumen of the appendix [62]. In fact, the only exception to conservative treatment in non-complicated appendicitis is the presence of an appendicolith. These patients present a high rate of failure and should not be treated conservatively [63–65].

Most surgeons agree that in case of non-complicated appendicitis, if operative management is decided, there are not differences regarding complications, between early and delayed treatment. Indeed, perforation of the appendix, small bowel obstruction, and surgical site infections did not seem to have higher rates in children who enter the operation room with a delay of a few hours, compared with those with an early appendicectomy [66–69]. On the other hand, complicated cases should be treated promptly, in order to avoid complications [70, 71]. According to the international guidelines, delayed appendicectomy, until 24 h after the presentation of symptoms, is safe and does not increase the risks of complications. Complicated cases should be treated with surgery no more than 8 h after admission to the hospital [36].

A debate exists on the optimal treatment in children with abscess or phlegmon. Meta-analyses have shown that although early appendectomy was associated with reduced length of hospital stay, children treated conservatively presented lower rates of complications and readmissions [72, 73]. Some believe that children treated with antibiotics and percutaneous drainage of an abscess can, also, avoid interval appendicectomy [74].

There is evidence that interval appendicectomy is not always necessary after successful conservative treatment of an abscess in the pediatric population. In a systematic review, the rate of recurrence after conservative management of complicated appendicitis in a mixed population of children and adults was 12%, and interval appendicectomy prevented the relapse of the disease in only one of eight patients [75]. The (CHINA) study, a multicenter, open-label, randomized controlled study at 19 specialist pediatric surgery centers, 17 of which were in the United Kingdom, one in Sweden, and one in New Zealand, showed that more than three-quarters of children could avoid appendectomy during early follow-up after successful NOM of an appendix mass. The proportion of children with recurrent acute appendicitis was 12%, and the proportion of children with severe complications related to interval appendicectomy was 6% [76]. Taking into consideration that in patients over 40 years, the risk of neoplasms is quite high (17%) [77], the international guidelines recommend a non-operative approach to children and young adults with complicated appendicitis, reserving appendectomy for patients who develop recurrence of the disease or recurrent symptoms [36].

The best non-operative treatment for uncomplicated appendicitis is the use of antibiotics. For simple appendicitis in adults, there is evidence of remission even without antibiotic therapy [78, 79], but no studies have been done for this purpose in children. The treatment with antibiotics for simple appendicitis follows the empiric regimens for non-critically ill patients with community-acquired intra-abdominal infections as advised by the 2017 WSES guidelines [80]. These are amoxicillin/clavulanate 6-hourly or ceftriaxone 24-hourly + metronidazole 6-hourly or cefotaxime 8-hourly + metronidazole 6-hourly. In patients with beta-lactam allergy, the antibiotic therapy should consist of ciprofloxacin + metronidazole 6-hourly or moxifloxacin 24-hourly. In patients at risk for infection with community-acquired ESBL-producing Enterobacteriaceae, ertapenem once a day or tigecycline in full dose initially and then every 12 h is the best option. Antibiotic therapy should consist of, at least, 48 h intravenous administration followed by oral intake for 7–10 days [36, 81].

8.2 Operative management

Surgical treatment has been the cornerstone for the definitive therapy of acute appendicitis. Claudius Amyand (1660–1740) performed in 1735 the first appendicectomy on an 11-year-old patient, although the initial diagnosis was right inguinal hernia (containing the perforated appendix) with a fistula to the right thigh [82]. Nowadays, laparoscopic operation is the first option in most medical centers, while robotic surgery seeming to be the next step in the minimal invasive surgical treatment.

Reviews of the literature have shown that a single dose of broad-spectrum antibiotics, given preoperatively, from 0 to 60 min before incision, is effective in decreasing the rate of complications, with no apparent difference concerning the severity of the inflammation of the appendix [36, 83, 84].

International guidelines suggest that for non-complicated appendicitis in children, postoperative therapy with antibiotics does not offer any advantage. For complicated cases, the most common regimen administered postoperatively is ampicillin, clindamycin (or metronidazole), and gentamicin for 7 days after surgery. Alternatively, ceftriaxone with metronidazole, or ticarcillin-clavulanate plus gentamicin, can be used [85]. In rates of efficacy, the use of metronidazole is superfluous, when broad-spectrum antibiotics such as aminopenicillins with β-lactam inhibitors or carbapenems and select cephalosporins are administered [86]. Some argue that double antibiotic therapy for pediatric patients has the same efficacy and is more cost-effective than triple therapy, but more evidence is needed [87]. It is widely accepted that children with complicated appendicitis can, safely, switch to oral antibiotics, as soon as 48 h after appendicectomy, without presenting increased rates of complications or readmission. Such regimen with oral antibiotics, also, showed no difference in length of stay but reduced hospital charges [36, 88–90].

Open appendicectomy is performed using, mostly, the McBurney incision. The laparoscopic technique is used with the same efficacy and safety for the removal of the appendix in children, regardless of the severity of the disease.

The laparoscopic technique follows the same basic principles of the open surgery, with the main difference being the cost, because of the special equipment. Furthermore, the cosmetic result is better with the laparoscopic method. It is widely accepted that laparoscopic appendectomy is associated with lower postoperative pain, lower incidence of complications, fewer days of hospitalization, and higher quality of life in children, regardless of the severity of the inflammation [36, 91, 92].

The argument on the use of drains in children with complicated appendicitis did not result in statistically significant differences between the drain and no drain groups in the rate of intra-abdominal abscesses, surgical site infections, and bowel obstruction. However, drains were statistically associated with an increased requirement for antibiotic and analgesic medication, fasting time, operative time, and length of hospital stay, and for that reason, are not recommended [36, 93].

9. Conclusion

In our times, the acute appendicitis is considered a disease with low morbidity, especially for the complicated cases, and mortality is minimal. Antibiotics, which used to play an important, but secondary role, especially in the postoperative treatment, nowadays have become the best option for the treatment of uncomplicated and certain complicated cases. The only problem remaining is the early and accurate diagnosis of the disease, which, even with various modern diagnostic modalities, remains still a challenge in the pediatric population.

Author details

George Sakellaris[1*], Xenophon Sinopidis[2], Konstantinos Zachos[3] and Ioannis Spyridakis[4]

1 Department of Pediatric Surgery, University General Hospital of Herakleion, Herakleion, Greece

2 Department of Pediatric Surgery, University of Patras School of Medicine, University General Hospital of Patras, Patras, Greece

3 Department of Pediatric Surgery, Pediatric Hospital of Patras, Patras, Greece

4 Department of Pediatric Surgery, Aristotle University of Thessaloniki School of Medicine, Papageorgiou General Hospital, Thessaloniki, Greece

*Address all correspondence to: georgesakellaris97@gmail.com

References

[1] Buschard K, Kjaeldgaard A. Investigation and analysis of the position. Fixation, length, and embryology of the vermiform appendix. Acta Chirurgica Scandinavica. 1973;**139**(3):293-298

[2] Ajmani ML, Ajmani K. The position, length, and arterial supply of vermiform appendix. Anatomischer Anzeiger. 1983;**153**:369-374

[3] Owen RL, Nemanic P. Antigen processing structures of the mammalian intestinal tract. Scanning Electron Microscope. 1978;**2**:367-378

[4] Maisel H. The position of the human vermiform appendix in fetal and adult age groups. Anatomical Record. 1960;**136**(3):385-391. DOI: 10.1002/ar.1091360305

[5] Sandler TW. Langman's Medical Embryology. 14th International ed. Philadelphia: Lippincott WW Publisher; 2018

[6] Parmar PD, Dave J, Vekariyia M, Pandya K. Study of variations in position of appendix in 100 operated case of appendicitis. International Journal of Health Sciences and Research. 2017;**7**(5):42-46

[7] Collins DC. 71000 human appendix specimens: A final report, summarizing forty years' study. American Journal of Proctology. 1963;**14**:365-381

[8] Babcock WW. Lumbar appendicitis, and lumbar appendectomy. Surgery, Gynecology and Obstetrics. 1946;**82**:414-416

[9] Fawcitt R. Appendix situated within thorax. British Journal of Radiology. 1948;**21**:523-525. DOI: 10.1259/0007-1285-21-250-523

[10] Arda IS, Senocak ME, Hicsönmez A. Duplication of the vermiform appendix: Case report and review of the literature. Pediatric Surgery International. 1992;**7**:221-222

[11] Wetzig NR. Diverticulosis of the vermiform appendix. Medical Journal of Australia. 1986;**145**(9):464-465. DOI: 10.5694/j.1326-5377.1986.tb113876.x

[12] Droga BW, Levine S, Baber JJ. Heterotopic gastric and esophageal tissue in the vermiform appendix. American Journal of Clinical Pathology. 1963;**40**:190-193. DOI: 10.1093/ajcp/40.2.190

[13] Viniol A, Keunecke C, Biroga T, Stadje R, Dornieden K, Bosner S, et al. Studies of the symptom abdominal pain—A systematic review and meta-analysis. Family Practice. 2014;**31**(5):517-529. DOI: 10.1093/fampra/cmu036

[14] Kang JY, Hoare J, Majeed A, Williamson RCN, Maxwell JD. Decline in admission rates for acute appendicitis in England. British Journal of Surgery. 2003;**90**:1586-1592. DOI: 10.1002/bjs.4363

[15] Ilves I, Fagerstrom A, Herzig KH, Juvonen P, Miettinen P, Paajanen H. Seasonal variations of acute appendicitis and nonspecific abdominal pain in Finland. World Journal of Gastroenterology. 2014;**20**(14):4037-4042. DOI: 10.3748/wjg.v20.i14.4037

[16] Bhangu A, Søreide K, Di Saverio S, Assarsson JH, Drake FT. Acute appendicitis: Modern understanding of pathogenesis, diagnosis, and management. Lancet. 2015;**386**(10000):1278-1287. DOI: 10.1016/S0140-6736(15)00275-5

[17] Grosfeld JL, O'Neil JA Jr, Goran AG, Fonkalsrud EW. Pediatric Surgery. 6th ed. Philadelphia: Mosby Publisher; 2006

[18] Livingston EH, Woodward WA, Sarosi GA, Haley RW. Disconnect between incidence of nonperforated and perforated appendicitis: Implications for pathophysiology and management. Annals of Surgery. 2007;**245**(6):886-892. DOI: 10.1097/01.sla.0000256391.05233.aa

[19] Cappendijk VC, Hazebroek FW. The impact of diagnostic delay on the course of acute appendicitis. Archives of Disease in Childhood. 2000;**83**(1):64-66. DOI: 10.1136/adc.83.1.64

[20] Lee SL, Stark R, Yaghoubian A, Shekherdimian A, Kaji A. Does age affect the outcomes and management of pediatric appendicitis? Journal of Pediatric Surgery. 2011;**46**(12):2342-2345. DOI: 10.1016/j.jpedsurg.2011.09.030

[21] Flum DR, Koepsel T. The clinical and economical correlates of misdiagnosed appendicitis: Nationwide analysis. Archives of Surgery. 2002;**137**(7):799-804. DOI: 10.1001/archsurg.137.7.799

[22] Birnbaum BA, Wilson SR. Appendicitis at the millennium. Radiology. 2000;**215**(2):337-348. DOI: 10.1148/radiology.215.2.r00ma24337

[23] Deng Y, Chang DC, Zhang Y, Webb J, Gabre-Kidan A, Abdullah F. Seasonal and day of the week variations of perforated appendicitis in US children. Pediatric Surgery International. 2010;**26**(7):691-696. DOI: 10.1007/s00383-010-2628-z

[24] Bickler SW, DeMaio A. Western diseases: Current concepts and implications for pediatric surgery research and practice. Pediatric Surgery International. 2007;**24**(3):251-255. DOI: 10.1007/s00383-007-2095-3

[25] Oestreich AE, Adelstein EH. Appendicitis as the presenting complaint in cystic fibrosis. Journal of Pediatric Surgery. 1982;**17**(2):191-194. DOI: 10.1016/s0022-3468(82)80212-1

[26] Brunicardi F, Andersen D, Billiar T, Dunn D, Hunter J, Pollock RE. Schwartz's Principles of Surgery. 8th ed. New York: McGraw-Hill Publisher; 2004

[27] Burkitt DP. The etiology of appendicitis. British Journal of Surgery. 1971;**58**(9):695-699. DOI: 10.1002/bjs.1800580916

[28] Gomes CA, Nunes TA, Chebli JMF, Soares C Jr, Gomes CC. Laparoscopic grading system of acute appendicitis: New insight for future trials. Surgical Laparoscopy Endoscopy and Percutaneous Techniques. 2012;**22**(5):463-466. DOI: 10.1097/SLE.0b013e318262edf1

[29] Brender DJ, Marcuse EK, Keopsell TD, Hatch EI. Childhood appendicitis: Factors associated with perforation. Pediatrics. 1985;**76**(2):301-302

[30] Monsalve S, Ellwanger A, Montedonico S. White blood cell count and C-reactive protein together remain useful for diagnosis and staging of acute appendicitis in children. South African Medical Journal. 2017;**107**(9):773-776. DOI: 10.7196/SAMJ.2017.v107i9.12206

[31] Vasquez-Rios G, Calixto-Aguilar L, Pajuelo R, Alarcon W. Thoracic empyema as rare complication of an appendicular mass: A case study and review of the literature. Case Reports in Pediatrics. 2018;**2018**:9640397. DOI: 10.1155/2018/9640397

[32] Almaramhy HH. Acute appendicitis in young children less than 5 years: Review article. Italian Journal of Pediatrics. 2017;**43**(1):15. DOI: 10.1186/s13052-017-0335-2

[33] Noh H, Chang SJ, Han A. The diagnostic values of preoperative laboratory markers in children with complicated appendicitis. Journal of the Korean Surgical Society. 2012;**83**(4):237-241. DOI: 10.4174/jkss.2012.83.4.237

[34] Benito J, Acedo Y, Medrano L, Barcena E, Perez Garay R, Arana Arri E. Usefulness of new and traditional serum biomarkers in children with suspected appendicitis. The American Journal of Emergency Medicine. 2016;**34**(5):871-876. DOI: 10.1016/j.ajem.2016.02.011

[35] Allister L, Bachur R, Glickman J, Horwitz B. Serum markers in acute appendicitis. The Journal of Surgical Research. 2011;**168**:70-75. DOI: 10.1016/j.jss.2009.10.02924

[36] Di Saverio S, Podda M, De Simone B, Ceresoli M, Augustin G, Gori A, et al. Diagnosis and treatment of acute appendicitis: 2020 update of the WSES Jerusalem guidelines. World Journal of Emergency Surgery. 2020;**15**(1):27. DOI: 10.1186/s13017-020-00306-3

[37] Dueholm S, Bagi P, Bud M. Laboratory aid in the diagnosis and prognosis of acute appendicitis: A blinded, prospective trial concerning diagnostic value of leukocyte count, neutrophil differential count and C-reactive protein. Diseases of the Colon and Rectum. 1989;**32**(10):855-859. DOI: 10.1007/BF02554555

[38] Douglas CD, Macpherson NE, Davidson PM, Sani JS. Randomised controlled trial of ultrasonography in diagnosis of acute appendicitis, incorporating the Alvarado score. British Medical Journal. 2000;**321**(7266):919-922. DOI: 10.1136/bmj.321.7266.919

[39] Kaiser S, Freckner B, Jorulf HK. Suspected appendicitis in children, us and CT—A prospective randomized study. Radiology. 2002;**233**(3):633-638. DOI: 10.1148/radiol.2233011076

[40] Love BE, Camelo M, Nouri S, Kriger D, Ludi D, Nguyen H. Ultrasound accuracy in diagnosing appendicitis in obese pediatric patients. American Surgeon. 2017;**83**(10):1063-1067

[41] Yi DY, Lee KH, Park SB, Kim JT, Lee NM, Kim H, et al. Accuracy of low dose CT in the diagnosis of appendicitis in childhood and comparison with USG and standard dose CT. Jornal de Pediatria. 2017;**93**(6):625-631. DOI: 10.1016/j.jped.2017.01.004

[42] Kinner S, Pickhardt PJ, Riedesel EL, Gill KG, Robbins JB, Kitchin DR, et al. Diagnostic accuracy of MRI versus CT for the evaluation of acute appendicitis in children and young adults. American Journal of Roentgenology. 2017;**209**(4):911-919. DOI: 10.2214/AJR.16.17413

[43] Dibble EH, Swenson DW, Cartagena C, Baird GL, Herliczek TW. Effectiveness of a staged US and unenhanced MR imaging algorithm in the diagnosis of pediatric appendicitis. Radiology. 2018;**286**(3):1022-1029. DOI: 10.1148/radiol.2017162755

[44] Zachos K, Fouzas S, Kolonitsiou F, Skiadopoulos S, Gkentzi D, Karatza A, et al. Prediction of complicated appendicitis risk in children. European Review for Medical and Pharmacological Sciences. 2021;**25**(23):7346-7353. DOI: 10.26355/eurrev_202112_27428

[45] Alvarado A. A practical score for the early diagnosis of acute appendicitis.

Annals of Emergency Medicine. 1986;**15**(5):557-564. DOI: 10.1016/s0196-0644(86)80993-3

[46] Andersson M, Kolodziej B, Andersson RE, STRAPPSCORE Study Group. Randomized clinical trial of Appendicitis Inflammatory Response score-based management of patients with suspected appendicitis: Appendicitis Inflammatory Response score-based management of suspected appendicitis. British Journal of Surgery. 2017;**104**(11):1451-1461. DOI: 10.1002/bjs.10637

[47] Scott AJ, Mason SE, Arunakirinathan M, Reissis Y, Kinross JM, Smith JJ. Risk stratification by the appendicitis inflammatory response score t95o guide decision-making in patients with suspected appendicitis. British Journal of Surgery. 2015;**1029**(5):563-537. DOI: 10.1002/bjs.9773

[48] Samuel M. Pediatric appendicitis score. Journal of Pediatric Surgery. 2002;**37**(6):877-881. DOI: 10.1053/jpsu.2002.32893

[49] Malik MU, Connelly TM, Awan F, Pretorius F, Ciuza-Castineira C, El Faedy O, et al. The RIPASA score is sensitive and specific for the diagnosis of acute appendicitis in a western population. International Journal of Colorectal Disease. 2017;**32**(4):491-497. DOI: 10.1007/s00384-016-2713-4

[50] Kulik DM, Uleryk EM, Maguire JL. Does this child have appendicitis? A systematic review of clinical prediction rules for children with acute abdominal pain. Journal of Clinical Epidemiology. 2013;**66**(1):95-104. DOI: 10.1016/j.jclinepi.2012.09.004

[51] Song CW, Kang JW, Kim JY. Different clinical features, and lower scores in clinical scoring systems for appendicitis in preschool children: Comparison with school age onset. Pediatric Gastroenterology, Hepatology and Nutrition. 2018;**21**(1):51-58. DOI: 10.5223/pghn.2018.21.1.51

[52] Macco S, Vrouenraets BC, de Castro SMM. Evaluation of scoring systems in predicting acute appendicitis in children. Surgery. 2016;**160**(6):1599-1604. DOI: 10.1016/j.surg.2016.06.023

[53] Scheller RL, Depinet HE, Ho ML, Hornung RW, Reed JL. Utility of pediatric appendicitis score in female adolescent patients. Academic Emergency Medicine. 2016;**23**(5):610-615. DOI: 10.1111/acem.12916

[54] Chung PHY, Dai K, Yang Z, Wong KKY. Validity of Alvarado score in predicting disease severity and postoperative complication in pediatric acute appendicitis. World Journal of Pediatric Surgery. 2019;**2**:e000003. DOI: 10.1136/wjps-2018-000003

[55] Sallinen V, Akl EA, You JJ, Agarwal A, Shoucair S, Vadvik PO, et al. Meta-analysis of antibiotics versus appendicectomy for non-perforated acute appendicitis. British Journal of Surgery. 2016;**103**(6):656-667. DOI: 10.1002/bjs.10147

[56] Georgiou R, Eaton S, Stanton MP, Pierro A, Hall NJ. Efficacy and safety of nonoperative treatment for acute appendicitis: A meta-analysis. Pediatrics. 2017;**139**(3):e20163003. DOI: 10.1542/peds.2016-3003

[57] Minneci PC, Mahida JB, Lodwick DL, Sulkowski JP, Nacion KM, Cooper JN, et al. Effectiveness of patient choice in nonoperative vs surgical management of pediatric uncomplicated acute appendicitis. JAMA Surgery. 2016;**151**(5):408-415. DOI: 10.1001/jamasurg.2015.4534

[58] Xu J, Adams S, Liu YC, Karpelowsky J. Nonoperative management in children with early acute appendicitis: A systematic review. Journal of Pediatric Surgery. 2017;**52**(9):1409-1415. DOI: 10.1016/j.jpedsurg.2017.05.003

[59] Huang L, Yin Y, Yang L, Wang C, Li Y, Zhou Z. Comparison of antibiotic therapy and appendectomy for acute uncomplicated appendicitis in children: A meta-analysis. JAMA Pediatrics. 2017;**171**(5):426-434. DOI: 10.1001/jamapediatrics.2017.0057

[60] Gorter RR, The S-MML, MAW G-S, Eker HH, Bakx R, van der Lee JH, et al. Systematic review of nonoperative versus operative treatment of uncomplicated appendicitis. Journal of Pediatric Surgery. 2017;**52**(8):1219-1227. DOI: 10.1016/j.jpedsurg.2017.04.005

[61] Kastritsi O, Sinopidis X, Barbagadakis S, Sakellaris S, Matzakanis G, Kastritsi ED, et al. Non-operative management of acute appendicitis in children: Single center, cohort study. Chirurgia (Turin). 2022;**35**(3):138-142. DOI: 10.23736/S0394-9508.21.05295-5

[62] Kessler U, Mosbahi S, Walker B, Hau EM, Cotton M, Peiry B, et al. Conservative treatment versus surgery for uncomplicated appendicitis in children: A systematic review and meta-analysis. Archives of Disease in Childhood. 2017;**102**(12):1118-1124. DOI: 10.1136/archdischild-2017-313127

[63] Svensson JF, Patkova B, Almström M, Naji H, Hall NJ, Eaton S, et al. Nonoperative treatment with antibiotics versus surgery for acute nonperforated appendicitis in children: A pilot randomized controlled trial. Annals of Surgery. 2015;**261**(1):67-71. DOI: 10.1097/SLA.0000000000000835

[64] Tanaka Y, Uchida H, Kawashima H, Fujiogi M, Takazawa S, Deie K, et al. Long-term outcomes of operative versus nonoperative treatment for uncomplicated appendicitis. Journal of Pediatric Surgery. 2015;**50**(11):1893-1897. DOI: 10.1016/j.jpedsurg.2015.07.008

[65] Lee SL, Spence L, Mock K, Wu JX, Yan H, DeUgarte D. Expanding the inclusion criteria for non-operative management of uncomplicated appendicitis: Outcomes and cost. Journal of Pediatric Surgery. 2018;**53**(1):42-47. DOI: 10.1016/j.jpedsurg.2017.10.014

[66] Serres SK, Cameron DB, Glass CC, Graham DA, Zurakowski D, Karki M, et al. Time to appendectomy and risk of complicated appendicitis and adverse outcomes in children. JAMA Pediatrics. 2017;**171**(8):740-746. DOI: 10.1001/jamapediatrics.2017.0885

[67] Almström M, Svensson JF, Patkova B, Svenningsson A, Wester T. In-hospital surgical delay does not increase the risk for perforated appendicitis in children: A single-center retrospective cohort study. Annals of Surgery. 2017;**265**(3):616-621. DOI: 10.1097/SLA.0000000000001694

[68] Gurien LA, Wyrick DL, Smith SD, Dassinger MS. Optimal timing of appendectomy in the pediatric population. Journal of Surgical Research. 2016;**202**(1):126-131. DOI: 10.1016/j.jss.2015.12.045

[69] Cameron DB, Williams R, Geng Y, Gosain A, Arnold MA, Guner YS, et al. Time to appendectomy for acute appendicitis: A systematic review. Journal of Pediatric Surgery. 2018;**53**(3):396-405. DOI: 10.1016/j.jpedsurg.2017.11.042

[70] Boomer LA, Cooper JN, Anandalwar S, Fallon SC, Ostlie D, Leys CM, et al. Delaying appendectomy

does not lead to higher rates of surgical site infections: A multi-institutional analysis of children with appendicitis. Annals of Surgery. 2016;**264**(1):164-168. DOI: 10.1097/SLA.0000000000001396

[71] Saluja S, Sun T, Mao J, Steigman SA, Oh PS, Yeo H, et al. Early versus late surgical management of complicated appendicitis in children: A statewide database analysis with one-year follow-up. Journal of Pediatric Surgery. 2018;**53**(7):1339-1344. DOI: 10.1016/j.jpedsurg.2017.09.012

[72] Fugazzola P, Coccolini F, Tomasoni M, Stella M, Ansaloni L. Early appendectomy vs. conservative management in complicated acute appendicitis in children: A meta-analysis. Journal of Pediatric Surgery. 2019;**54**(11):2234-2241. DOI: 10.1016/j.jpedsurg.2019.01.065

[73] Vaos G, Dimopoulou A, Gkioka E, Zavras N. Immediate surgery, or conservative treatment for complicated acute appendicitis in children? A meta-analysis. Journal of Pediatric Surgery. 2019;**54**(7):1365-1371. DOI: 10.1016/j.jpedsurg.2018.07.017

[74] Luo C-C, Cheng K-F, Huang C-S, Lo H-C, Wu S-M, Huang HC, et al. Therapeutic effectiveness of percutaneous drainage and factors for performing an interval appendectomy in pediatric appendiceal abscess. BMC Surgery. 2016;**16**:72. DOI: 10.1186/s12893-016-0188-4

[75] Darwazeh G, Cunningham SC, Kowdley GC. A systematic review of perforated appendicitis and phlegmon: Interval appendectomy or wait-and-see? American Surgeon. 2016;**82**(1):11-15

[76] Hall NJ, Eaton S, Stanton MP, Pierro A, Burge DM, CHINA study collaborators and the Paediatric Surgery Trainees Research Network. Active observation versus interval appendicectomy after successful non-operative treatment of an appendix mass in children (CHINA study): An open label, randomised controlled trial, lancet. Gastroenterology and Hepatology. 2017;**2**(4):253-260. DOI: 10.1016/S2468-1253(16)30243-6

[77] Mällinen J, Rautio T, Grönroos J, Rantanen T, Nordstrom P, Savolainen G, et al. Risk of appendiceal neoplasm in periappendicular abscess in patients treated with interval appendectomy vs follow-up with magnetic resonance imaging: 1-year outcomes of the peri-appendicitis acuta randomized clinical trial. JAMA Surgery. 2019;**154**(3):200-207. DOI: 10.1001/jamasurg.2018.4373

[78] Sippola S, Grönroos J, Sallinen V, Rautio T, Nordstrom P, Rantanen T, et al. A randomised placebo-controlled double-blind multicentre trial comparing antibiotic therapy with placebo in the treatment of uncomplicated acute appendicitis: APPAC III trial study protocol. BMJ Open. 2018;**8**(11):e023623. DOI: 10.1136/bmjopen-2018-023623

[79] Salminen P, Sippola S, Haijanen J, Nordström P, Rantanen T, Rautio T, et al. Antibiotics versus placebo in adults with CT-confirmed uncomplicated acute appendicitis (APPAC III): Randomized double-blind superiority trial. British Journal of Surgery. 2022:znac086. DOI: 10.1093/bjs/znac086

[80] Sartelli M, Chichom-Mefire A, Labricciosa FM, Hardcastle T, Abu-Zidan FM, Adesunkanmi AK, et al. The management of intra-abdominal infections from a global perspective: 2017 WSES guidelines for management of intra-abdominal infections. World Journal of Emergency Surgery. 2017;**12**:29. DOI: 10.1186/s13017-017-0141-6

[81] Podda M, Cillara N, Di Saverio S, Lai A, Feroci F, Luridiana G, et al. Antibiotics-first strategy for uncomplicated acute appendicitis in adults is associated with increased rates of peritonitis at surgery, a systematic review with meta-analysis of randomized controlled trials comparing appendectomy and non-operative management with antibiotics. The Surgeon. 2017;**15**(5): 303-314. DOI: 10.1016/j.surge.2017.02.001

[82] Panagidis A, Sinopidis X, Zachos K, Alexopoulos V, Vareli A, Varvarigou A, et al. Neonatal perforated Amyand's hernia presenting as an enterocutaneous scrotal fistula. Asia Journal of Surgery. 2015;**38**(3):177-179. DOI: 10.1016/j.asjsur.2014.03.001

[83] Andersen BR, Kallehave FL, Andersen HK. Antibiotics versus placebo for prevention of postoperative infection after appendicectomy. Cochrane Database of Systematic Reviews. 2005;(3):CD001439. DOI: 10.1002/14651858.CD001439.pub2

[84] Wu W-T, Tai F-C, Wang P-C, Tsai M-L. Surgical site infection and timing of prophylactic antibiotics for appendectomy. Surgical Infections. 2014;**15**(6):781-785. DOI: 10.1089/sur.2013.167

[85] Lee SL, Islam S, Cassidy LD, Abdullah F, Arca MJ, 2010 American Pediatric Surgical Association Outcomes and Clinical Trials Committee. Antibiotics and appendicitis in the pediatric population: An American pediatric surgical association outcomes and clinical trials committee systematic review. Journal of Pediatric Surgery. 2010;**45**(11):2181-2185. DOI: 10.1016/j.jpedsurg.2010.06.038

[86] Shang Q, Geng Q, Zhang X, Guo C. The efficacy of combined therapy with metronidazole and broad-spectrum antibiotics on postoperative outcomes for pediatric patients with perforated appendicitis. Medicine. 2017;**96**(47):e8849. DOI: 10.1097/MD.0000000000008849

[87] Dreznik Y, Feigin E, Samuk I, Kravarusic D, Baazov A, Levy I, et al. Dual versus triple antibiotics regimen in children with perforated acute appendicitis. European Journal of Pediatric Surgery. 2018;**28**(6):491-494. DOI: 10.1055/s-0037-1606847

[88] Arnold MR, Wormer BA, Kao AM, Klima DA, Colavita PD, Cosper GH, et al. Home intravenous versus oral antibiotics following appendectomy for perforated appendicitis in children: A randomized controlled trial. Pediatric Surgery International. 2018;**34**(12):1257-1268. DOI: 10.1007/s00383-018-4343-0

[89] Sujka JA, Weaver KL, Sobrino JA, Poola A, Gonzalez KW, St Peter SD. Efficacy of oral antibiotics in children with post-operative abscess from perforated appendicitis. Pediatric Surgery International. 2019;**35**(3):329-333. DOI: 10.1007/s00383-018-4424-0

[90] Loux TJ, Falk GA, Burnweit CA, Ramos C, Knight C, Malvezzi L. Early transition to oral antibiotics for treatment of perforated appendicitis in pediatric patients: Confirmation of the safety and efficacy of a growing national trend. Journal of Pediatric Surgery. 2016;**51**(6):903-907. DOI: 10.1016/j.jpedsurg.2016.02.057

[91] Yu M-C, Feng Y, Wang W, Fan W, Cheng H-T, Xu J. Is laparoscopic appendectomy feasible for complicated appendicitis? A systematic review and meta-analysis. International Journal of Surgery. 2017;**40**:187-197. DOI: 10.1016/j.ijsu.2017.03.022

[92] Zhang S, Du T, Jiang X, Song C. Laparoscopic appendectomy in children with perforated appendicitis: A meta-analysis. Surgical Laparoscopy, Endoscopy, and Percutaneous Techniques. 2017;**27**(4):262-266. DOI: 10.1097/SLE.0000000000000411

[93] Aneiros Castro B, Cano I, García A, Yuste P, Ferrero E, Gomez A. Abdominal drainage after laparoscopic appendectomy in children: An endless controversy? Scandinavian Journal of Surgery. 2018;**107**(3):197-200. DOI: 10.1177/1457496918766696

Chapter 3

Neglected Appendicitis

Venkatachalam Raveenthiran, Nagarajan Darun and Shanmugam Shobini

Abstract

Prompt diagnosis and surgical excision of inflamed appendix vermiformis is a goal that is often elusive in clinical practice. An overall delay more than 36 hours from the onset of symptoms can be defined as neglected appendicitis. Factors responsible for delay may be pre-hospital versus in-hospital, physician centered versus patient centered, medical versus socioeconomic and modifiable versus unmodifiable. Consequences of neglected diagnosis or treatment may be perforation, general peritonitis, adhesive bowel obstruction, prolonged ileus, mass formation, appendicular and metastatic abscesses, pyelephlebitis, stump appendicitis and fecal fistula. Non-operative antibiotic treatment followed by interval appendicectomy is recommended in neglected appendicitis to avoid collateral surgical injury to inflamed cecum. If surgical excision is unavoidable in acute phase, mucosa coring salvage (MUCOSAL) appendicectomy is preferred. It is important to recognize that clinical neglect is not the same as criminal neglect.

Keywords: appendicitis, appendicectomy, acute abdomen, delayed diagnosis, neglected treatment, medicolegal issues, imaging studies

1. Introduction

Appendicitis is one of the most common surgical emergencies throughout the world [1, 2]. Its incidence is 100 per 100,000 person years [2]. Of the 675,000 children visiting emergency department (ED) for abdominal pain, about 80,000 (11%) underwent appendectomy [3]. It is now well established that prompt diagnosis and early surgical removal of the inflamed appendix is paramount for avoiding morbidity and mortality. However, this goal often remains elusive in clinical practice.

The diagnosis of appendicitis is missed in 4.8 to 15% of children and in 5 to 23% of adults during their first visit to ED [3, 4]. In some series the diagnostic error was as high as 53% [5]. Accurate differential diagnosis remains a challenge even in the era of modern imaging [3]. Despite routine use of CT scan and ultrasound the frequency of misdiagnosis persisted at 15% over 2 decades (**Figure 1**) [6, 7]. However, a few studies have noted a drop in misdiagnosis from 25–6% when a CT scan is used [8]. There are some indications that the rate of missed diagnoses is steadily falling in recent times, perhaps due to increased experience with modern imaging methods. The rate of missed diagnosis was 28% in 1990 [9], 7% in 1993 [10], and 4.8% in 2013 [3]. Even if a moderate diagnostic error of 5% is acknowledged, its cumulative impact will be huge. For example, in 2019, globally 17.7 million patients were newly diagnosed with appendicitis

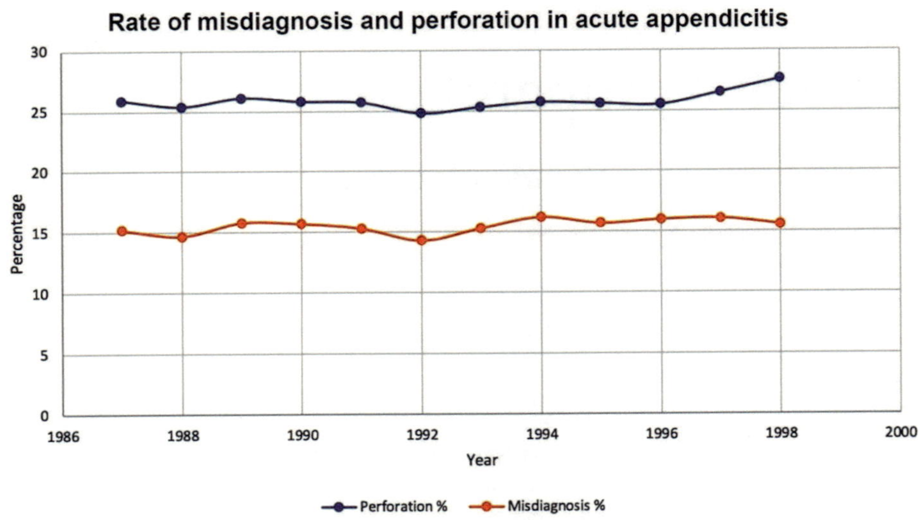

Figure 1.
Graph showing the absence of any improvement in the misdiagnosis rate of acute appendicitis over a decade. (Constructed based on the data from: Flum DR, et al. JAMA 2001).

and by estimate 880,000 patients would have been misdiagnosed [11]. Consequences of diagnostic delay are deferred treatment, prolonged hospitalization, increased morbidity, higher mortality and undue escalation of the cost of health care [12].

2. Definition

Delay or neglect in the diagnosis or treatment of appendicitis can be measured either directly or indirectly by surrogate markers such as perforation rates and mass formation. But there is no universally agreed definition as to what can be termed as 'neglected appendicitis'. Goyal et al. defined it as missed diagnosis when the patient had visited an ED at least once within the preceding 7 days of correct diagnosis [13]. Some authors fixed the cutoff point as 48 hours [14, 15]. Others disagreed with these high cutoff points as the incidence of perforation in children rose from 10% at 18 hours to 44% at 36 hours of symptom-onset [16]. The frequencies of Grade 1 to 4 appendicitis were 94%, 0%, 3%, and 3%, respectively if the total delay (symptom onset to operation) was within 12 hours; while the respective frequencies of disease severity changed to 60%, 7%, 27%, and 6% between 48 and 71 hours and to 54%, 7%, 26%, and 13% if the interval is longer than 71 hours [17].

Several studies and meta-analyses have shown that a brief in-hospital delay within 24 hours of admission is not associated with increased complication rates [18–21]. Contrary to this other authors have noted complication rates increased from 6% with an in-hospital delay of 6 hours to 14% at 12–18 hours [22, 23]. It is also noted that pre-hospital delays are more detrimental than in-hospital delays, probably because of the protection offered by antibiotics in admitted patients [5].

Considering the foregoing facts, inflamed appendix vermiformis can be defined as 'neglected appendicitis' if its diagnosis or treatment is delayed for more than 36 hours from the onset of symptoms [24, 25]. We do not find any practical advantage of further splitting the cut off points into pre-hospital delay of 24 hours and in-hospital delay of 12 hours.

It is important not to confuse 'criminal neglect' with 'clinical neglect'; the former is contrived, ill-intended and punishable by court of law while the later is mostly inadvertent, circumstantial or even deliberately professed for the well being of patients. 'Clinical neglects' are often due to inherent limitations of medical science, complexities of human pathophysiology or socioeconomic factors. It is important that clinical neglects be reduced by training, education and welfare measures rather than by punishments, lest it will backfire on the society.

3. Factors of delay

Delay may occur in the diagnosis or treatment of acutely inflamed appendix and the former may occur in pre-hospital setting or after admission to a hospital. Factors of delay may be patient-related or physician-related. Some of them are modifiable while others are non-modifiable.

3.1 Age of patients

Extremes of age are more liable for pre-hospital diagnostic delays [9, 26, 27]. Dependency on caretakers for hospital visits, inability to accurately express symptoms (either because of dementia or immaturity), absence of economic freedom and altered pain perception are common in both infants and elderly [26]. The younger the child, the more difficult is an accurate diagnosis. None of the neonatal appendicitis was diagnosed preoperatively and a mean delay of 8 days (5–11 days) is not unusual in this age group [28]. Age less than 30 years [5] and that above 55 years [29] are found to be associated with significant pre-hospital delays. A mean delay of 3 days (2–5 days) is usual in elderly patients [30].

3.2 Sex of patients

Several authors [5, 29] found male gender at a higher risk of pre-hospital delay while others [14, 31] found females more vulnerable. Gender bias and discrimination of girl children is not unknown in many underdeveloped countries. Besides this, delay in adult females is also partly due to non-classical symptoms and closely mimicking differential diagnosis such as ectopic pregnancy [31].

3.3 Rural and remote population

Access to health care facility is often a challenge for rural population [5, 32, 33] and remote inhabitants such as those of Himalayan high altitude [34]. In Australia, rural families had to travel a mean distance of 50 km for consulting a physician and it resulted in a mean delay of 42 hours [35]. Transportation delay was as much as 3 to 7 days in rural Africa. The mean ambulance transport time from district hospital to referral hospital was as much as 4.9 hours [33]. Rural people treated at an urban facility have more frequent perforations than rural people treated at local rural hospitals. This is suggestive of the detrimental effect of delayed transportation [36]. Even in countries with air ambulance service, significant delay is attributed to physician disagreement on transfers and data connectivity [37].

Rural people are also more likely to have superstitious beliefs which prevent them from seeking timely medical help [38]. Some of the primitive tribes exhibit trust deficit with urban hospitals and modern medicine. For example, the cultural safety and hostility of Maori tribe of New Zealand and Jarawa tribe of Andaman Islands remains a problem [35]. It was also suggested that increased complication in rural children may be due to more severity of the disease per se rather than due to transportation delay [39]. There are some data showing that the urban–rural gap is now started narrowing in some countries [40].

3.4 Race and ethnicity

Perforated appendicitis is more common in Black children due to delayed treatment as compared to that of Hispanics [41]. Black children with appendicitis are subjected to less frequent imaging than non-Hispanic Whites. This may be due to racial discrimination or due to insurance status [13]. Maori children of Australia had more perforation (28.9%) than White children (19%) [39]. Some authors deny the existence of any racial difference or discrimination [42].

3.5 Duration of symptoms

Those with shorter duration of symptoms at initial visit are more likely to be misdiagnosed. About 69% of those who visited ED within 24 hours of symptom onset were misdiagnosed [43]. This paradox can be explained by the atypical nature of evolving symptoms that overlap with many other non-surgical disorders. In delayed cases, diagnosis becomes self-evident by the established signs of complications such as peritonitis [22].

3.6 Weak-end and wee-hour presentations

Patients who present in midnight and wee-hours are often misdiagnosed [43]. They typically undergo less investigations and stay for shorter period in ED. Non-availability of the services of senior consultants, and physical exhaustion of ED personnel could contribute to diagnostic delays in wee-hours. Circadian variation in surgeons' ability to diagnose appendicitis was, however, denied by Danish researchers [44]. Children who presented on Mondays had more risk of perforation [45]. Interestingly, the odds of perforation were 30% higher in those who presented in working hours (9 am – 3 pm) than in those who presented in wee hours [46]. These paradoxes can be explained by the challenges of transportation in weekends and wee hours.

3.7 Self medications

As much as 23% of pre-hospital delay was due to self medications and home remedies tried by patients [47]. The risk is especially more if father is the caregiver [48]. Over the counter sale of antibiotics, which is common in many southeast Asian and African countries, partially mask the symptoms thereby contributes to diagnostic delays [48]. Interestingly, in Nigeria, antibiotic self-medication did not adversely affect outcome despite causing significant pre-hospital delay [49]. Beneficial effect of antibiotics in controlling infection appears to compensate the detrimental effect of delayed hospital admission. Early empirical usage of non-steroidal analgesics but not opioid analgesics was found to cause delay in seeking medical help [50].

3.8 Season

In a rural population, complicated appendicitis was more common in winter (75%) than in other seasons (33%) [51]. Interestingly, appendicitis is generally accepted to be more common in summers than in winters. For every increase of 5.56°C of environmental temperature, the incidence of appendicitis increases by 1.3% [52]. Therefore the observed seasonal difference in complications may be attributed to the challenges of transportation in winter.

3.9 Educational and socioeconomic status

Pre-hospital delay is significantly reduced in educated population. Physicians and other medical workers develop perforation less often than general population [53]. It was suggested that insurance status rather than actual socioeconomic status of patients influences the diagnostic and therapeutic delay. For obvious reasons, uninsured patients often present late and they undergo less investigation than insured citizens [53, 54]. However, data from one American center denied any correlation between the frequency of appendicular perforation and educational level, income or insurance status [42].

3.10 Pandemics

Lockdown of covid-19 pandemic posed enormous challenges in accessing health care services and caused inordinate delay in treatment [55–57]. Frequency of perforation (38 vs. 21%), gangrene (23 vs. 16%) and peri-appendicular abscess (5 vs. 1%) were higher during pandemic time than during the preceding year [55]. Number of consultations for acute appendicitis decreased by 20% as compared to pre-pandemic times [56]. Pre-hospital delay as long as 2 days [57] was suggesting either transportation difficulties or reluctance of patients in attending hospitals. On the other hand, co-existence of Covid-19 caused severe conflicts in therapeutic decision making and thereby contributed to in-hospital delay. Exhaustion of hospital resources, risk of spreading covid-19 infection to the surgical team, unknown implications of operating upon a Covid-19 patient and financial hardship of lockdown frequently resulted in postponement of appendicectomy. Most often patients were managed non-operatively with antibiotics although it is clearly undesirable at other times [56]. Interestingly, a children's hospital in Spain did not find any significant difference in pre-hospital symptom duration, laboratory investigation, hospital stay, intensive care admissions or diagnostic errors during the pandemic [58].

3.11 Coexisting diseases

Not infrequently presence of coexisting diseases causes delay in the management of appendicitis by masking or mimicking the classical symptoms, by posing conflicts of priority in intervention, by interfering with imaging and laboratory diagnosis and by preventing access to health care services. For example, inability to express symptoms, altered pain perception and dependency on care takers to reach hospital are common in neurological disorders such as dementia, schizophrenia, mental retardation, deaf mutism and cerebral palsy [59]. However, a Taiwanese study refuted any association between mental disorders and therapeutic delays in acute appendicitis [60]. Altered perception of pain due to visceral neuropathy, associated nephropathy, atypical symptoms that overlap with ketoacidosis are known to cause significant diagnostic delay in diabetics [61]. Obesity is known to interfere with clinical diagnosis and surgical approach of acute appendicitis [62].

Aortic aneurysm, myocardial infarction, Henoch-Schonlein Purpura, myelodysplasia, leukemia, lymphoma, carcinoid tumors, cecal carcinoma, Kawasaki disease, gastroenteritis, typhoid fever and measles are frequently know to coexist with appendicitis and cause serious therapeutic dilemma. Adverse effects of drugs used to treat coexisting diseases such as chemotherapy of cancers, hypertension and end-stage renal disease pose serious therapeutic dilemma thereby cause considerable delay in doing appendicectomy [63]. Appendicitis secondary to blunt injury of abdomen (post-traumatic appendicitis) is invariably mistaken for hemoperitoneum; however, fortunately therapeutic interventions are not delayed in such patients [64].

3.12 Mimicking diseases

Although most of the diagnostic delays occur at the level of primary care physicians, specialist consultants at tertiary care centers are not immune to this. Physician related diagnostic delays are often due to the dilemma caused by overlapping symptoms of acute appendicitis with that of other abdominal emergencies. The list of differential diagnosis of acute appendicitis is very long including several infectious diseases, genitourinary pathologies, metabolic disorders and malignancies [65]. Recently, Covid-19 related MISC (Multisystem Inflammatory Syndrome in Children) was reported to mimic appendicitis [66]. Better imaging and liberal use of laboratory investigations may avoid diagnostic errors and in-hospital delays.

3.13 Pregnancy

Typical clinical presentation of appendicitis is seen in only 50 to 60% of pregnant women [67]. Approximately 50% of appendicitis occur in the second trimester [67]. The frequency of perforated appendicitis in the first, second and third trimester are 8.7%, 12.5%, and 26.1% respectively [67]. The symptoms of early appendicitis, such as nausea and vomiting, are also seen in the morning sickness of pregnancy. The normal febrile response to appendicular infection may be blunted in pregnancy [68]. Classical tenderness at McBurney's point may be absent in pregnancy as the gravid uterus causes cephalad or posterior displacement of the appendix. Lower quadrant pain of the second trimester produced by traction on the suspensory ligaments of the uterus, a phenomenon known as round ligament pain, may be confused with appendicular pain [69]. Choice of imaging is also restricted in pregnancy as CT scan cannot be used due to concerns of radiation exposure. Gravid uterus overlying the appendix will also interfere with adequate sonographic imaging. Finally, laboratory tests such as leucocytosis that are typical of appendicitis are commonly seen during normal pregnancy. However, pain in the right lower quadrant of the abdomen remains the cardinal feature of appendicitis in pregnancy. Ectopic pregnancy or uterine contractions many also mimic or coexist with appendicular pain. Fetal loss occurs in 3–5% of uncomplicated appendicitis which increases to 20% in perforated cases. Laparotomy especially in first and third trimester carries the risk of abortion or premature delivery [70]. Because of these reasons, a subconscious reluctance is often noted among surgeons in diagnosing acute appendicitis and operating upon pregnant women.

3.14 Physician of first contact

Patients consulting an appropriate specialist during first visit are less likely to be misdiagnosed than those who consult general physicians or family practitioners [71, 72]. The later more often tend to diagnose medical disorders and treat conservatively than surgeons who swiftly decide on surgical operation [73]. Physicians who omit imaging or WBC counts are more likely to miss the diagnosis [4]. When the initial physician missed the diagnosis, the perforation rate increased from 20 to 31% [4].

3.15 Choice of initial imaging

Patients who received only an abdominal x-ray rather than a ultrasonography or a CT scan are more likely to be misdiagnosed [74]. Presence of local ileus often precludes penetration of ultrasound waves leading to non-visualization of the appendix. In doubtful cases, laparoscopy may be used both as a diagnostic as well as a therapeutic tool. Diagnostic accuracy of laparoscopy approaches 98% and it picks up even cases that are missed in CT scan or sonography [75]. MRI is an alternative for accurate diagnosis but it requires interpretation by an imaging expert [76].

3.16 Anatomical location of appendix

Clinical features of acute appendicitis are partly determined by the anatomical position of the organ. Among orthotopic appendices, retrocecal position notoriously masks local tenderness and presents with backache [77]. Pre- or post- ileal appendices may be mistaken for gastroenteritis and pelvic appendix for urinary tract infection [78].

Correct diagnosis is invariably missed on first ED visit if the appendix is ectopically located. Subhepatic appendicitis is often mistaken for cholecystitis [79]. Only 50% of patients had a correct preoperative diagnosis when the appendix was located on the left-iliac fossa or epigastrium as it is in situs inversus or midgut malrotation [80]. Intrathoracic appendix associated with diaphragmatic hernia may mimic acute chest pain [81]. Herniated appendix into the scrotum (Amyand hernia) may be mistaken for epididymo-orchitis or testicular torsion [82]. In all these cases diagnosis is seldom made on first ED visit.

3.17 In-hospital therapeutic delays

Despite admission to hospital, surgical intervention is often delayed for several reasons which include diagnostic dilemma, waiting for emergency operation slot and interruption of therapeutic plans by co-existing diseases [83]. Fortunately in-hospital delays as long as 24 hours are found to be safer than pre-hospital delays [84]. This is because of the administration of intravenous antibiotics under watchful eyes [85]. If an appendectomy is done on the day of admission, the perforation rate was 28.8% while it increased to 33.3% on day 2 and 78.8% by day 8 [12].

Inordinate delay in the diagnosis and intervention may also happen in postoperative appendicitis that develops in 0.1% of patients undergoing major surgery [86]. Diagnosis will be extremely difficult if the original surgery was a laparotomy. It may occur 5–31 days after the primary operation and its diagnosis is delayed 12 hours to 8 days [86]. These patients required hospitalization for as long as 80 days.

4. Prevention of diagnostic delays

Diagnostic delays are significantly reduced when the primary physician performs the triad of leukocyte count, C-reactive protein and ultrasonography [87]. Several scoring systems have also been proposed to minimize diagnostic ambiguities. Alvarado score in adults and Samuel score in children are very popular [88]. There are also computer driven algorithms such as Eskelinen Scoring and online Pediatric Appendicitis Risk Calculator (PARC) [Kharbanda - https://www.mdcalc.com]. Role of artificial intelligence in improving the diagnostic accuracy is currently under validation [89, 90]. Resource allocation to improve ambulance services and hospital infrastructure may avoid in-hospital delays but their implementation will continue to be a challenge especially in underdeveloped countries.

5. Consequences of neglected appendicitis

5.1 Perforation

With delay in diagnosis or treatment, appendicular inflammation progresses to cause perforation [91]. Pathogenic mechanisms of perforation are diverse including inflammatory suppuration of the appendicular wall, gangrene secondary to thrombosis of the appendicular artery and rupture due to built-up intraluminal pressure of fermented gases or pent-up secretions [92]. Perforation causes spillage of fecal matter and infected luminal contents in to the peritoneal cavity. Consequences of the spillage depend up on the pattern of perforation: (1) In *tardy perforation*, as it is in the case of non-obstructive appendicitis that is treated partially with antibiotics, omentum and adjacent bowel loops get stuck to the appendix thereby effectively sealing the infected material from spreading through-out the general peritoneal cavity. This adhesion complex is known as appendicular mass or phlegmon. (2) *Swift perforation* occurs either because of high bacterial virulence or due to poor host-defense. In the absence of adhesion formation, spillage occurs into the general peritoneal cavity leading to generalized peritonitis. Frequency of perforation is influenced by therapeutic delay while the pattern of perforation is determined by other factors [93]. For example, poor development of omentum in infants prevents mass formation and favors earlier onset of general peritonitis than adults. About 30% of acute appendicitis in children results in uncontained perforation (range 20–74%) and it reaches 100% in infants below 1-year of age [94]. Luminal obstruction of fecolith causes violent rupture by the built-up pressure (**Figure 2**). Debility of old age, immune compromised states and diabetes tilt the balance towards general peritonitis. Conversely, anatomical padding of the appendix as it in the case of retrocecal and pelvic positions favors mass formation. Adhesions as a result of previous abdominal operations also help in containing the spillage.

5.2 General peritonitis

General peritonitis occurs mostly as a complication of appendicular perforation (**Figure 3**). But it can also occur in simple uncomplicated appendicitis. Clinical features of general peritonitis are unmistakable [95]. Extensive diagnostic work-up is irrelevant at this stage. Emergency laparotomy not only provides diagnostic solution but also the life saving therapy. *Escherichia coli* and mixed anaerobes are frequently isolated from the peritoneal cavity [96]. Primary appendicectomy with peritoneal

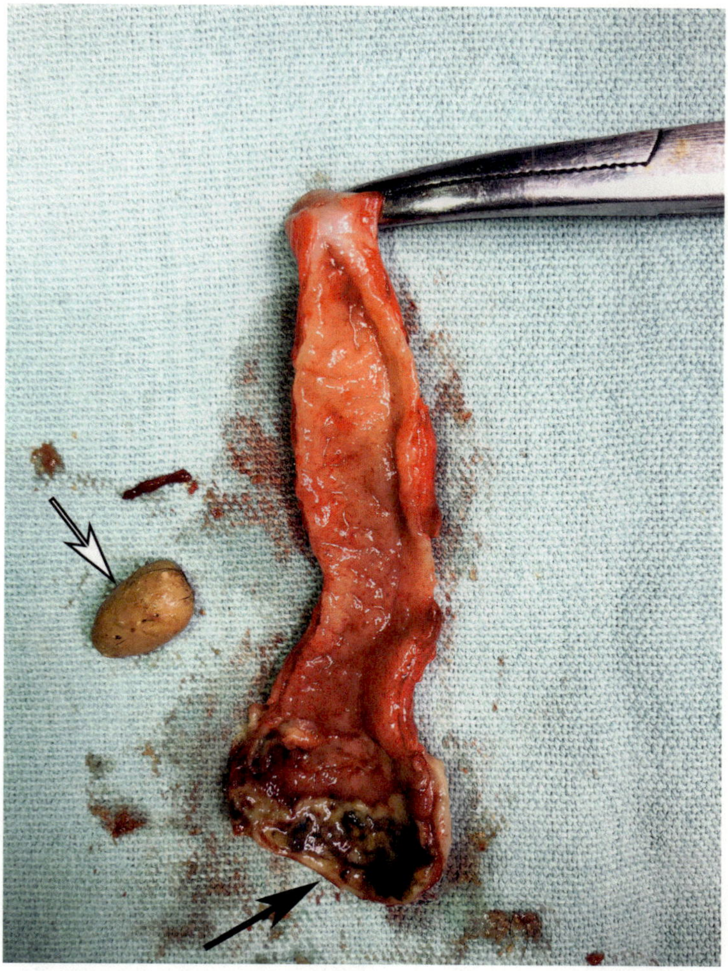

Figure 2.
Fecolith (white arrow) causing necrosis and perforation (black arrow) of the tip of inflamed appendix (the appendicular blow-out).

lavage and drains are recommended in general peritonitis. However, a recent study found increased complications with usage of peritoneal drains [97]. Open surgery as compared to laparoscopic appendicectomy was found to be associated with increased risk of bacteremia, endotoxemia and systemic inflammation [98]. Appendicular peritonitis in patients undergoing peritoneal dialysis poses special therapeutic problems. Fortunately mortality of well managed appendicular peritonitis is less than 1% even in resource poor countries [99].

5.3 Prolonged ileus

Prolonged ileus as a sequela of appendicular peritonitis is seen in 1–5% of patients [100]. Ileus may be due to bacterial toxins, electrolyte imbalance (hypokalemia), inflammatory edema or adverse effects of medications. More importantly, postoperative mechanical obstruction should not be mistaken for paralytic ileus. Consequences of such misdiagnosis are devastating as paralytic ileus is treated expectantly while

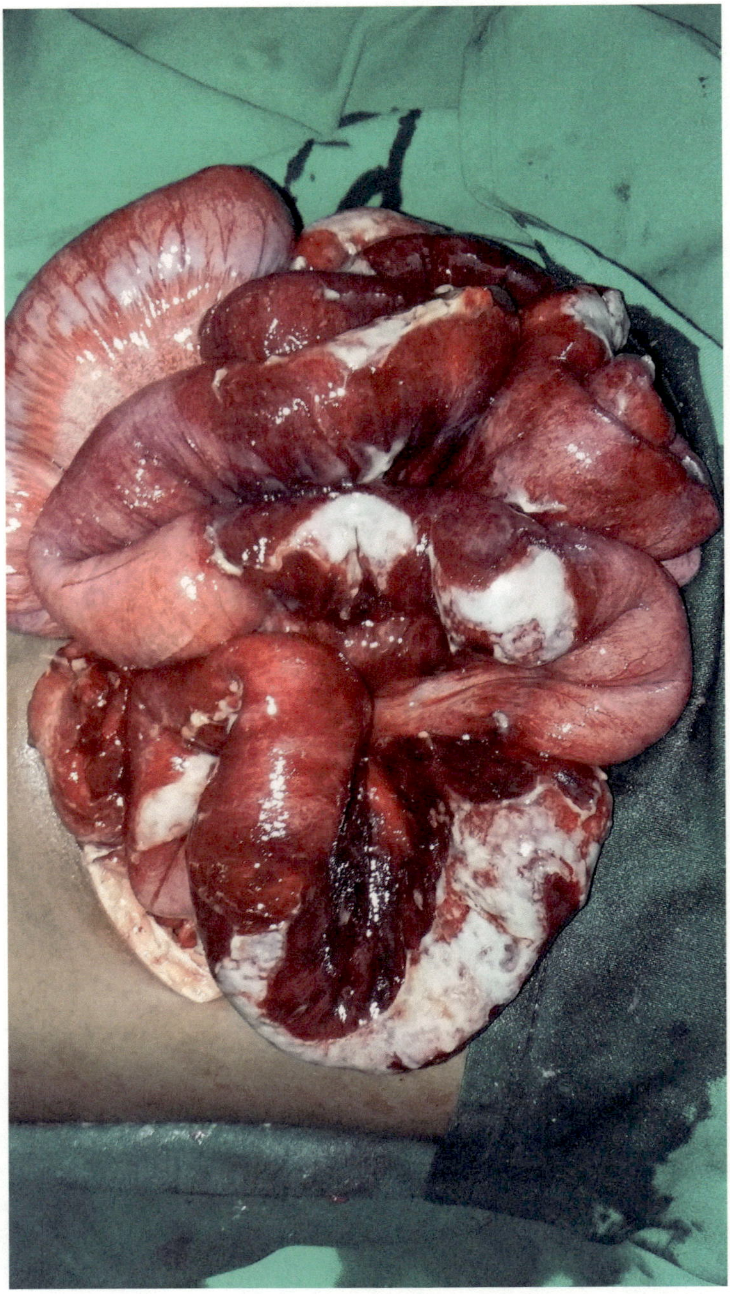

Figure 3.
Perforated appendicitis with general peritonitis.

mechanical obstruction necessitates prompt re-laparotomy. The duration of ileus is proportional to the duration, severity and extent of peritonitis. Some amount of ileus is common in the first 72 hours of appendicectomy. But if it prolongs beyond 72 hours it should be considered pathological [101]. The senior author has seen ileus persisting for 15 days. Prokinetic agents such as metoclopromide may be useful in stimulating the paralyzed bowel.

5.4 Appendicular mass (phlegmon)

Appendicular mass is composed of ileum, cecum, mesentery, fallopian tube and omentum that are adherent to the inflamed appendix. It may occur with or without perforation. Appendicular mass is usually formed after 72 hours from the onset of symptoms [102]. Attempted appendicectomy at this stage is more likely to cause collateral damage to the cecum and the adherent bowel which are rendered friable by inflammation (**Figure 4**). Therefore, general recommendation is to treat appendicular mass conservatively with Ochsner Sherren regimen [103, 104]. Presence of fecolith, leukocyte count >15,000/mm [3], bandemia, CT scan showing extension of mass beyond the limits of the right lower quadrant are factors that contraindicate non-operative management of appendicular mass.

Further fate of the mass is determined by the virulence of infection, presence of perforation and success of antimicrobial treatment. If medical treatment is successful, the appendicular mass will resolve. On the other hand, progression of suppurative infection transforms the mass into an abscess.

5.5 Appendicular abscess

Appendicular abscess is collection of pus within appendicular mass due to ongoing infection [105]. It may occur with or without perforation. It may be intraperitoneal, retroperitoneal or pelvic depending on the anatomical position of the appendix. In addition to administration of broad spectrum antibiotics, the pus has to be surgically drained. Temptation to do appendicectomy at the time of abscess drainage is better desisted as adherent bowel loops will be friable leading to operative injury [106, 107].

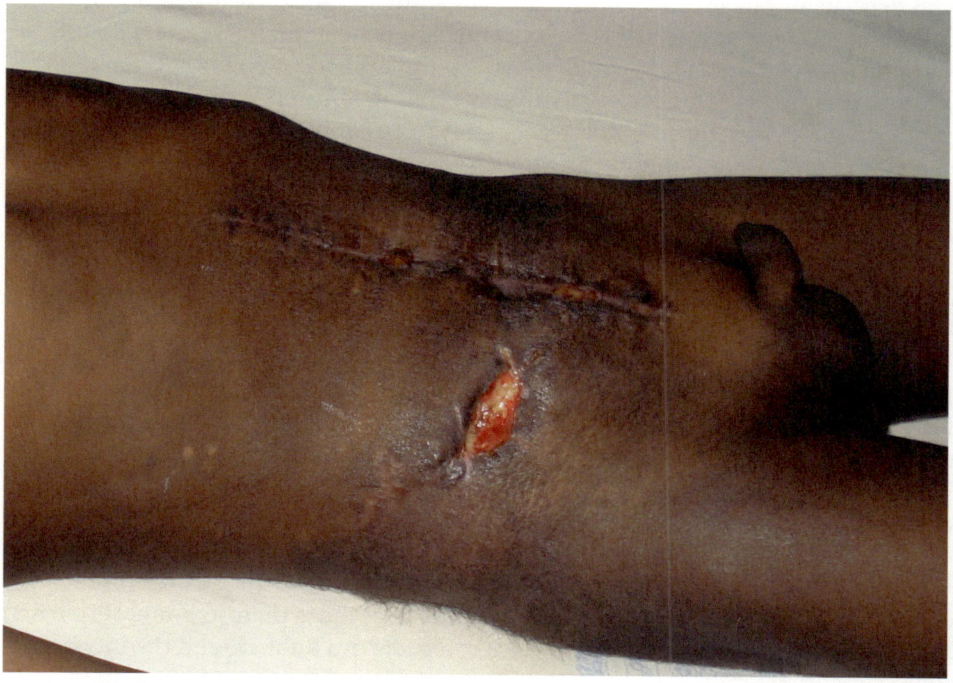

Figure 4.
Fecal fistula following attempted appendicectomy in a boy with appendicular mass.

Even intraperitoneal abscesses can be drained by extraperitoneal approach as the adhesions effectively seals the abscess cavity from rest of the peritoneal cavity. Pelvic abscess can be drained per rectally.

If proper treatment is neglected, appendicular abscess may rupture into the peritoneal cavity causing general peritonitis, into hollow viscera causing internal fistula or may rupture externally causing fecal fistula. Spread of infection may also result in intra-peritoneal or metastatic abscesses, meningitis, endocarditis, myocarditis and Systemic Inflammation Response Syndrome (SIRS).

5.6 Metastatic abscess

Direct or hematogenous spread of infection from the appendix is known to cause metastatic abscesses in adjacent or distant organs. Anatomical drainage of the appendicular vein into the portal vein facilitates lodging of septic emboli in the liver parenchyma causing liver abscess [108]. Direct fistulation of appendix into the liver has also been reported [109]. Seepage of infected fluid through the patent processes vaginalis or femoral canal can result in scrotal or right thigh abscess respectively [110, 111]. Rupture of liver abscess into pleural space or hematogenous spread of infection may cause empyema or lung abscess [112]. Metastatic abscesses of CNS [113], spleen [114], kidneys [115] are also known to complicate neglected appendicitis.

5.7 Fecal fistula

Apart from iatrogenic cecal injuries during appendicectomy, spontaneous rupture or surgical drainage of appendicular abscess may also result in fecal fistula. Such fistulae may be internal or external. Appendico-vesical fistula (n = 120) is the most common type of internal fistula complicating appendicitis [116]; followed by appendico-rectal [117], appendico-ileal [116], appendico-colic [118] fistulae. External appendico-cutaneous fistulae may occur in loin [119], thigh, groin [120] or umbilicus [121]. Usually, fecal matter and pus from suppurated appendicitis dissect their way externally and present as simple soft tissue abscess. Upon surgical drainage of such unsuspected abscess, fecal fistula will ensue. Multiple aerobes and anaerobes of the fecal fistula may cause extensive necrotizing fasciitis - also known as Meleney's ulcer [122]. Co-existing actinomycosis, Crohn's disease, luminal obstruction by tumors or fecolith and tuberculous enteritis favors the development of fecal fistula complicating appendicitis [123].

Fistulogram or CT scan is essential for diagnosing fecal fistula (**Figure 5**). Prompt appendicectomy, with or without cecal resection, is necessary to cure the fistula. However, appendico-colic fistulae may be managed conservatively and they require surgical intervention only if symptomatic.

5.8 Intestinal adhesive obstruction

Small bowel adhesion leading to intestinal obstruction is not an uncommon sequela of appendicitis if overall therapeutic delay is more than 36 hours (**Figure 6**) [124]. Adhesions of inflamed appendix may also form a knot around the intestinal loops (appendicular knotting) causing strangulation and gangrene of small bowel [125].

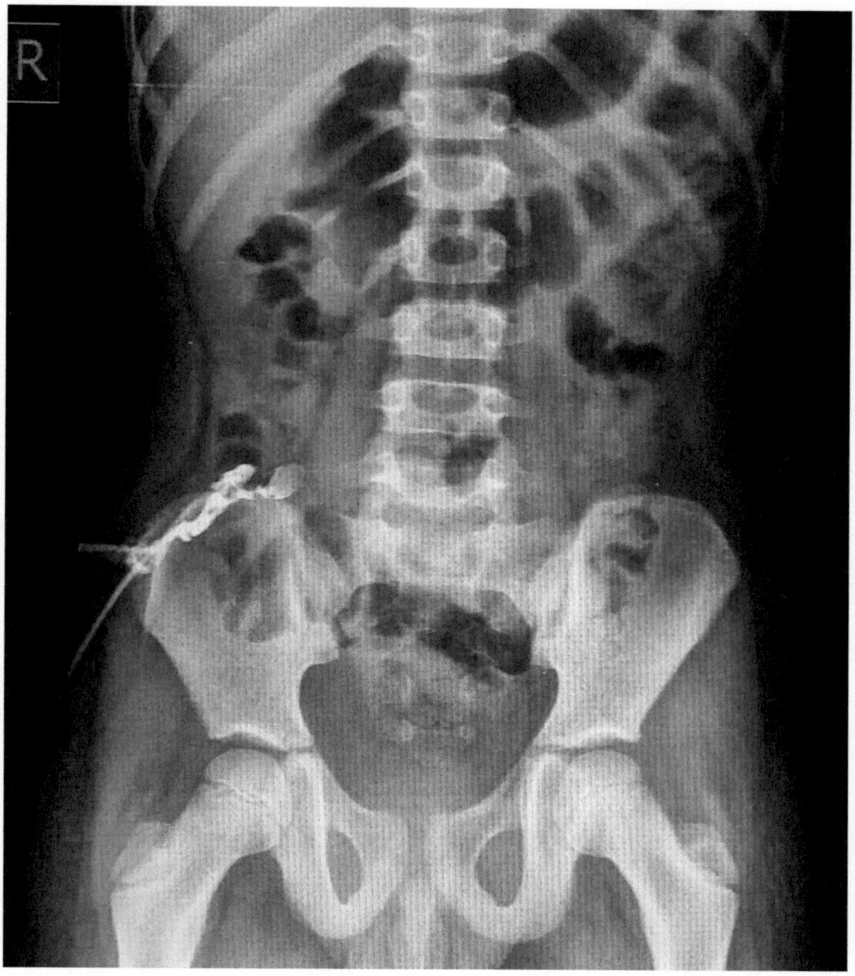

Figure 5.
Fistulogram delineating appendico-cutaneous fistula.

5.9 Stump appendicitis

Inadvertent failure to do complete excision leaves behind a stump of the appendix that may subsequently get inflamed. It occurs in 0.25% of appendicectomy and it is more common with laparoscopic excision [126]. Factors responsible for incomplete appendicectomy are lack of tactile feedback during laparoscopy, extensive plastering of appendix to cecal wall thereby obscuring its anatomical limits and inexperience on the part of surgeon. History of prior appendicectomy often precludes stump appendicitis from being considered as a differential diagnosis of recurrent abdominal pain. Although excision of the stump was sufficient in 94%, about 6% patients required extended resection of cecum to address the problem [126].

5.10 Pyelephlebitis

Septic thrombophlebitis of the portal vein is one of the most serious complications of neglected appendicitis. Its incidence is 0.05% in simple appendicitis and it

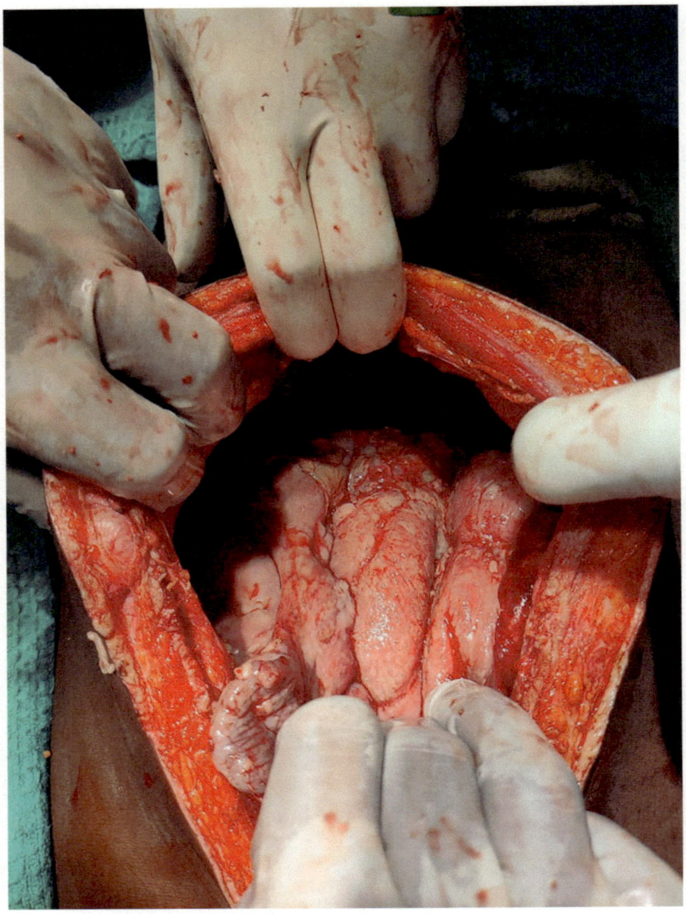

Figure 6.
Frozen peritoneum following perforated appendicitis. It is an extensive form of bowel adhesions and peritoneal plastering.

dramatically increases to 3% in delayed cases [127]. This rare complication should be suspected in appendicitis if the patient presents with a high fever and mild jaundice. Doppler or CT scan will demonstrate thrombus in the portal vein. Despite aggressive treatment, hepatic abscesses (50%) and mortality (30 to 50%) are not uncommon. Survivors of acute pyelephlebitis may develop portal hypertension, cavernous transformation of the portal vein and esophago-gastric varices.

6. Choice of imaging in neglected appendicitis

Ultrasound is the diagnostic investigation of choice in early as well as neglected appendicitis [128]. It is simple, easily available, cost-effective and is without radiation hazard. However, overlying bowel gas may interfere with the transmission of ultrasound waves and preclude sonographic visualization of the organ in case of appendicular mass or retrocecal appendicits. In such cases, contrast enhanced CT (CECT) scan will be useful [129]. Presence of peri-appendicular fluid or pus collection, extraluminal or intramural gas, appendicular wall enhancement defect,

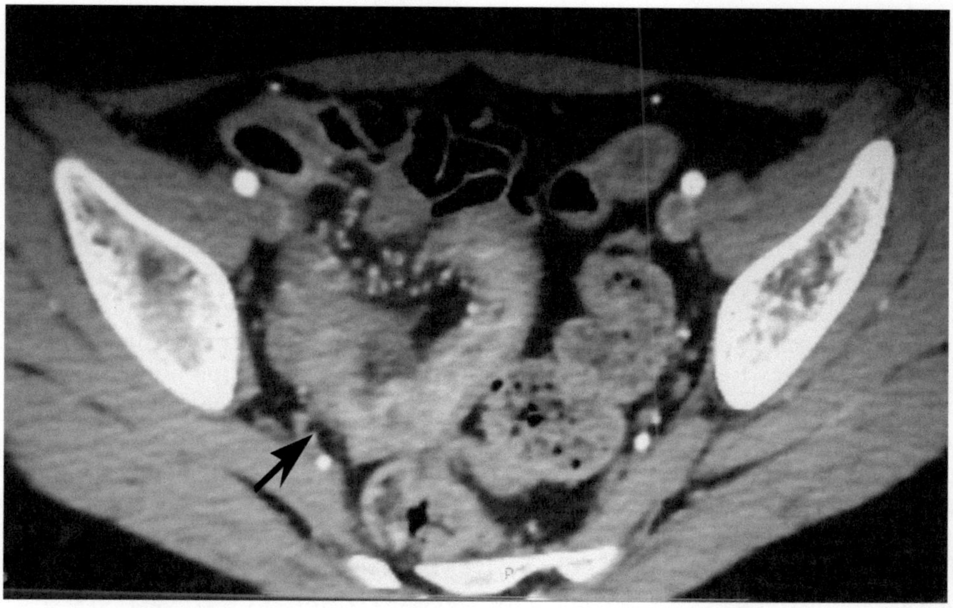

Figure 7.
Contrast enhanced CT scan showing appendicular mass (arrow).

Imaging modality	Sensitivity	Specificity	Positive predictive value	Negative predictive value
Ultrasound (USG)	32–86%	60–93%	42–60%	80–93%
CT scan (CECT)	28–95%	71–100%	74%	93%
MRI	37–75%	77–92%	58%	86%
USG + CECT	30–67%	85–97%	70%	84%

** Neglected appendicitis includes complicated pathologies such as perforation, phelgmon and abscess. These figures are compiled from the meta-analysis of Bom et al. [128]. CECT – Contrast enhanced computed tomography, MRI-Magnetic resonance imaging.*

Table 1.
*Comparative efficacy of imaging modalities in diagnosing neglected appendicitis.**

peri-appendiceal fat stranding, ascites, local ileus and free floating or luminal fecolith are the features that differentiate neglected (complicated) appendicitis from simple appendicitis (**Figure 7**) [129]. MRI does not appear to offer any added advantage over CECT in neglected appendicitis. It is often suggested that conditional CT scan combined with ultrasonography is beneficial (**Table 1**).

7. Management of neglected appendicitis

7.1 Ochsner Sherren (non-operative) regimen

Although Claudius Amyand performed the first successful appendicectomy in 1735 CE, its popularity catapulted only after 1902 CE when King Edward VII underwent dramatic surgical drainage of appendicular abscess just before his coronation.

It had even become fashionable among English nobility to request for prophylactic appendicectomy. Therefore, no one thought of non-surgical management of inflamed appendix. Ironically in the same year (1902 CE) Albert Ochsner of Chicago first suggested that conservative management followed by interval appendicectomy is better than immediate operation of appendicular mass. Later in 1905 James Sherren of London modified and popularized Ochsner's treatment which came to be known as 'Ochsner Sherren' regimen.

Ochsner Sherren regimen [130] consists of high Fowler's (propped-up) position, strict monitoring of pulse and vomiting, only sips of plain water orally for 5 days followed by gradual restarting of semisolid diet, absolute ban on enema and avoiding any drugs especially those that could mask pain, vomiting or diarrhea. The size of the appendicular mass is marked on the skin and its size-reduction is monitored. Patients with hyperesthesia, age less than 5 years, uncertainty of diagnosis, general peritonitis and those who had received purgatives are exempted from this treatment. The regimen is abandoned in favor of laparotomy if pulse rate increases, if pain persists, if the lump is not getting smaller after 5 days of treatment, if the lump becomes visible when viewed tangentially, if the mass becomes fluctuant, if the temperature is swinging or if a pelvic abscess is palpated. Hamilton Bailey typically described the indication of Ochsner-Sherren regimen as "appendicitis that is too late for the early operation and too early for the late operation" [130]. In Bailey's series, out of the 73 patients treated non-operatively only one died. This impressively low mortality of 1.4% was considered a wonder in pre-antibiotic era [130]. However, keeping up with the popular trend, an interval appendicectomy was advised after 8 weeks.

Despite the discovery of antibiotics in 1920s and their wide availability in 1940s, Ochsner-Sherren regimen remained popular until 1980s just because it was endorsed by none other than the venerable Hamilton Bailey and McNeil Love in their universally popular textbook, 'Short Practice of Surgery'. Bailey and Love's advice was backed by lot of wisdom. They advised routine appendicectomy if the duration of symptoms was less than 48 hours beyond which Ochsner Sherren regimen was recommended. This is because attempted separation of appendix from adhesions would result in fecal fistula and death due to operative injury to friable bowel loops.

Appropriateness of Ochsner Sherren regimen was reexamined in the era of newer antibiotics and advanced surgical techniques. Results are conflicting: some studies [131–133] claim cost effectiveness and low complication rates with non-operative treatment while others [134, 135] found a clear advantage of immediate appendicectomy even in delayed cases. A meta-analysis noted increased complication with surgical management and less efficacy with exclusive antibiotic therapy [135]. A Turkish study found the length of hospital stay was longer in conservative group while the cost of care was increased in operated patients. However, morbidity and mortality were similar in both groups [131]. Taiwanese surgeons found shorter duration of fever (2.7 vs. 8.0 days), delayed oral feeds (4.4 vs. 1.8 days), higher complication rate (33 vs. 17%) among emergently operated children as compared to those who were treated conservatively [132].

Interest in conservative treatment is recently rekindled by Covid-19 pandemic. Due to concerns of covid-19 infection, appendicitis was mostly treated non-operatively during the pandemic [136, 137]. Interestingly, this time, the scope of non-operative treatment is extended even to early cases and is not restricted to just appendicular phelgmon as it was originally proposed by Ochsner and Sherren. It is even suggested that conservative management may become the choice of treatment of all acute appendicitis irrespective of diagnostic or therapeutic delays [138].

7.2 Interval appendicectomy

Following conservative treatment recurrence of appendicitis was noted in 24% of children at a mean follow up of 16 months [139] and in 19% of adults at 33 months [140]. This prompted the recommendation of elective interval appendicectomy. However its indispensability was recently questioned [102, 141–143]. A meta-analysis found increased complications with early appendicectomy while interval appendicectomy incurred more cost [105].

The only feared complication of acute appendicitis is its rupture and life-threatening fecal peritonitis. However, there are some data to suggest that successive episodes of recurrent appendicitis are progressively less severe with negligible risk of perforative peritonitis [144]. This is because the inflamed appendix heals by fibrosis and peri-appendiceal adhesions effectively contain any spillage. With each episode of inflammation the appendix gets progressively fibrosed and eventually becomes a fibrous cord. Therefore, it appears prudent to forego interval appendicectomy in favor of wait-and watch or repeated conservative management. However, we would recommend elective interval appendicectomy in selected cases such as remote rural population, more than 2 attacks that require hospitalization, children below 8 years and presence of serious co-existing diseases.

7.3 Mucosal appendicectomy

Deliberate excision of appendix by dissecting the appendicular mass, though not desirable, has to be occasionally performed for various reasons. Sometimes, even after surgical drainage of appendicular abscess, sepsis will not abate because of ongoing

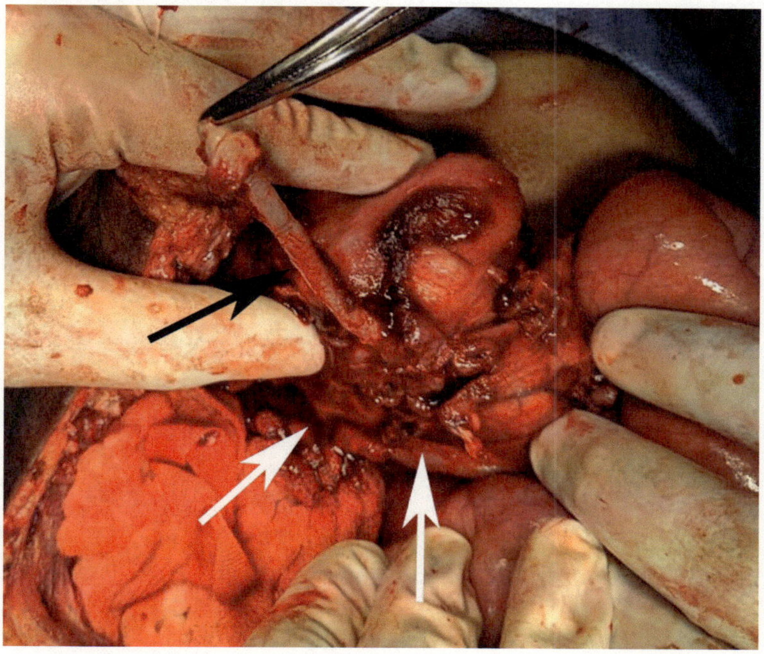

Figure 8.
MUCOSAL appendicectomy. Mucosal tube of appendix (black arrow) is being dissected off its muscular cuff (white arrows).

appendicular inflammation or leakage of fecal matter into the abscess cavity. In such cases appendicectomy is inevitably essential to control sepsis. However dense adhesions make surgical approach hazardous. Attempted separation of appendix from adjacent structures is sure to invite operative injury and fecal fistula. To avoid this trouble, Raveenthiran has described a new technique called MUCOSAL appendicectomy (**Figure 8**) [145].

The concept was first hinted in 2006 by Rangarajan et al. and in 2020 Raveenthiran described the technique in great detail and named it as 'MUCOSAL appendicectomy'. The nomenclature is an acronym of 'mucosa coring salvage appendicectomy'. This technique is also variously known as 'subserosal', 'submucosal' or 'trans-mesoappendicular' appendicectomy [145]. In this technique, the appendix is exposed by gentle finger dissection of adhesions (**Figure 9**). However, no attempt is made to isolate it from cecum or other adherent structures. A longitudinal sero-muscular incision is made and the mucosal tube is gently dissected off the muscular cuff similar to the dissections of Soave's endorectal pull-through operation or Lilly's operation for choledochal cyst. The dissected mucosal tube is ligated at its base and the redundant portion is excised. The seromuscluar cuff is left undisturbed. As appendicitis is essentially a disease of mucosa, removal of mucosal layer rather than the whole appendix is sufficient to prevent further attacks. Contrary to expectations, dissections in submucosal plane do not cause significant bleeding, as the tiny blood vessels are occluded either by thrombosis or by inflammatory edema. Therefore, it is safe to perform MUCOSAL appendicectomy even in the presence of disseminated intravascular coagulation syndrome.

7.4 Role of laparoscopy

The role of minimally invasive surgery (laparoscopy) in neglected appendicitis is slowly evolving [146, 147]. Long incisions of open surgery, that are required for better surgical access of adherent appendix, can be negated in laparoscopy. Thus, the risks of wound site infection, incisional hernia, hospital stay are low with laparoscopic approach. On the other hand, pneumoperitoneum of laparoscopy is thought to cause

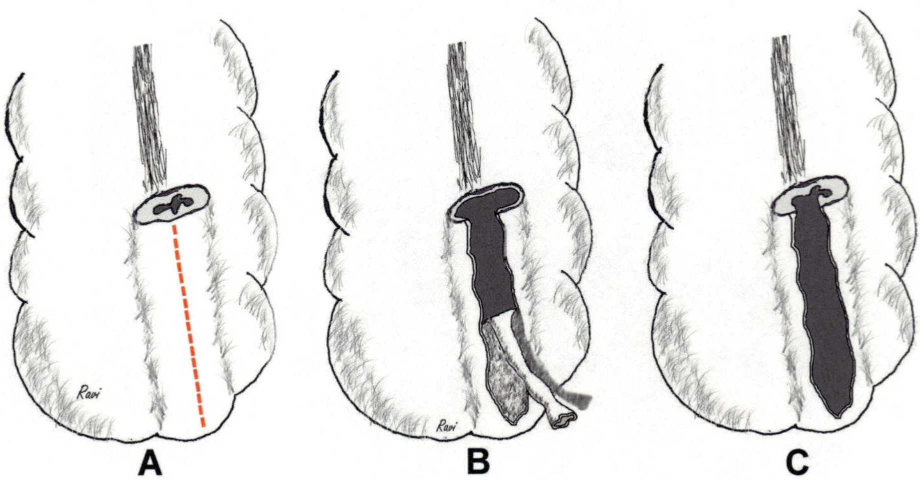

Figure 9.
Diagrammatic illustration of the principles of MUCOSAL appendicectomy. (A - Seromuscular incision over the appendix adherent to cecum; B - Dissection of mucosal tube; C - Completion of MUCOSAL appendicectomy leaving behind the seromuscular cuff).

widespread dissemination of infection which would have otherwise remained limited to the right lower quadrant. For this reason, intra-abdominal abscesses are more common with laparoscopic appendicectomies [148].

8. Outcome of neglect

Death due to appendicitis is now rare and it is 0.07 to 0.1% [149] or 4 per million-population [150]. However, with a pre-hospital delay of 1 week or more, mortality increases to 5.6% [151]. Death rate reaches as high as 20% when delay is combined with co-morbidities such as cardiovascular diseases [149]. Maternal mortality increases by fivefold and fetal loss by twofold when delay occurs in appendicitis of pregnancy [152]. Premature labor or abortion occurs in 15% of neglected appendicitis [152].

9. Medico-legal issues of neglect

Missed or delayed diagnosis of acute appendicitis is the second most common cause of legal litigations against emergency physicians [153]. Liberal use of multi-detector computed tomography and magnetic resonance imaging does not appear to reduce the risk of misdiagnosis [154]. Therefore, meticulous history and physical examination remains indispensible even in this era of advanced technology. Nearly 50% of litigations are related to post-operative complications, 20% to misdiagnosis and 7% to intra-operation mishaps [155]. In litigious cases patient-related delay ranges from 12 hours to 45 days while physician-related delay ranges from 2 to 430 hours. Interestingly, physician-related delays are relatively safer and shorter than patient-related delays [155]. Therefore, in case of diagnostic uncertainty, it is better to admit the patient for in-hospital monitoring. With passage of time, diagnosis of many cases that were initially ambiguous will become self-evident by the evolution of classical features [155].

Despite prompt diagnosis and meticulous execution of therapeutic interventions morbidity and mortality of appendicitis cannot be completely annulled. Unexpected or unfortunate outcomes prompt aggrieved patients to legally challenge the quality of care. In such cases physician may take defense in obtaining informed consent, recording the diagnostic difficulties and therapeutic dilemmas and by doing necessary investigations. Defense may also be taken by emphasizing lack of motives and ill intensions.

Author details

Venkatachalam Raveenthiran*, Nagarajan Darun and Shanmugam Shobini
Department of Pediatric Surgery, Government Cuddalore Medical College, Chidambaram, India

*Address all correspondence to: vrthiran@gmail.com

References

[1] Galai T, Beloosesky OZ, Scolnik D, et al. Misdiagnosis of acute appendicitis in children attending the emergency department: The experience of a large, tertiary care pediatric hospital. European Journal of Pediatric Surgery. 2017;**27**:138-141

[2] Ferris M, Quan S, Kaplan BS, et al. The global incidence of appendicitis: A systematic review of population-based studies. Annals of Surgery. 2017;**266**:237-241

[3] Naiditch JA, Lautz TB, Daley S, et al. The implications of missed opportunities to diagnose appendicitis in children. Academic Emergency Medicine. 2013;**20**:592-596

[4] Graff L, Russell J, Seashore J, et al. False-negative and false-positive errors in abdominal pain evaluation: Failure to diagnose acute appendicitis and unnecessary surgery. Academic Emergency Medicine. 2000;**7**:1244-1255

[5] Alyhari Q, Ahmed F Sr, Nasreldin M, et al. Prehospital delay and its associated factors in Sudanese patients presenting with acute appendicitis at a teaching hospital. Cureus. 2022;**14**:e23036

[6] Flum DR, Morris A, Koepsell T, Dellinger EP. Has misdiagnosis of appendicitis decreased over time? A population-based analysis. JAMA. 2001;**286**:1748-1753

[7] Flum DR, McClure TD, Morris A, Koepsell T. Misdiagnosis of appendicitis and the use of diagnostic imaging. Journal of the American College of Surgeons. 2005;**201**:933-939

[8] Naoum JJ, Mileski WJ, Daller JA, et al. The use of abdominal computed tomography scan decreases the frequency of misdiagnosis in cases of suspected appendicitis. American Journal of Surgery. 2002;**184**:587-589; discussion 589-90. DOI: 10.1016/s0002-9610(02)01086-3

[9] Rothrock SG, Skeoch G, Rush JJ, Johnson NE. Clinical features of misdiagnosed appendicitis in children. Annals of Emergency Medicine. 1991;**20**:45-50

[10] Reynolds SL. Missed appendicitis in a pediatric emergency department. Pediatric Emergency Care. 1993;**9**:1-3

[11] Yang Y, Guo C, Gu Z, et al. The global burden of appendicitis in 204 countries and territories from 1990 to 2019. Clinical Epidemiology. 2022;**14**:1487-1499

[12] Papandria D, Goldstein SD, Rhee D, et al. Risk of perforation increases with delay in recognition and surgery for acute appendicitis. The Journal of Surgical Research. 2013;**184**:723-729

[13] Goyal MK et al. Racial and ethnic disparities in the delayed diagnosis of appendicitis among children. Academic Emergency Medicine. 2021;**28**:949-956

[14] Kambouri K, Aggelidou M, Deftereos S, et al. What are the risk factors responsible for the delay in diagnosis of acute appendicitis in children? Eleven-year research from a single institution. Folia Med (Plovdiv). 2019;**61**:389-396

[15] Nomura O, Ishiguro A, Maekawa T, et al. Antibiotic administration can be an independent risk factor for therapeutic delay of pediatric acute appendicitis. Pediatric Emergency Care. 2012;**28**:792-795

[16] Narsule CK, Kahle EJ, Kim DS, et al. Effect of delay in presentation on rate of perforation in children with appendicitis. The American Journal of Emergency Medicine. 2011;**29**:890-893

[17] Ditillo MF, Dziura JD, Rabinovici R. Is it safe to delay appendectomy in adults with acute appendicitis? Annals of Surgery. 2006;**244**:656-660

[18] Kim SH, Park SJ, Park YY, Choi SI. Delayed appendectomy is safe in patients with acute nonperforated appendicitis. International Surgery. 2015;**100**:1004-1010

[19] Abou-Nukta F, Bakhos C, Arroyo K, et al. Effects of delaying appendectomy for acute appendicitis for 12 to 24 hours. Archives of Surgery. 2006;**141**:504-507

[20] Yardeni D, Hirschl RB, Drongowski RA, et al. Delayed versus immediate surgery in acute appendicitis: Do we need to operate during the night? Journal of Pediatric Surgery. 2004;**39**:464-469

[21] Bhangu A, (United Kingdom National Surgical Research Collaborative). Safety of short, in-hospital delays before surgery for acute appendicitis: Multicentre cohort study, systematic review, and meta-analysis. Annals of Surgery. 2014;**259**:894-903

[22] Ashkenazi I, Zeina AR, Olsha O. In-hospital delay of surgery increases the rate of complicated appendicitis in patients presenting with short duration of symptoms: A retrospective cohort study. European Journal of Trauma and Emergency Surgery. 2022;**48**:3879-3886

[23] Kovler ML, Pedroso FE, Etchill EW, et al. Prolonged In-hospital time to appendectomy is associated with increased complicated appendicitis in children. Annals of Surgery. 2022;**275**:1200-1205

[24] Bickell NA, Aufses AH, Rojas M, Bodian C. How time affects the risk of rupture in appendicitis. Journal of the American College of Surgeons. 2006;**202**:401-406

[25] Eldar S, Nash E, Sabo E, et al. Delay of surgery in acute appendicitis. American Journal of Surgery. 1997;**173**:194-198

[26] Cibert-Goton V, Kung VWS, McGuire C, et al. Functional and anatomical deficits in visceral nociception with age: A mechanism of silent appendicitis in the elderly? Pain. 2020;**161**:773-786

[27] Omling E, Salö M, Saluja S, et al. Nationwide study of appendicitis in children. The British Journal of Surgery. 2019;**106**:1623-1631

[28] Raveenthiran V. Neonatal appendicitis (part 1): A review of 52 cases with abdominal manifestation. Journal of Neonatal Surgery. 2015;**4**(1):4

[29] Augustin T, Cagir B, Vandermeer TJ. Characteristics of perforated appendicitis: Effect of delay is confounded by age and gender. Journal of Gastrointestinal Surgery. 2011;**15**:1223-1231

[30] Lunca S, Bouras G, Romedea NS. Acute appendicitis in the elderly patient: Diagnostic problems, prognostic factors and outcomes. Romanian Journal of Gastroenterology. 2004;**13**:299-303

[31] McGann Donlan S, Mycyk MB. Is female sex associated with ED delays to diagnosis of appendicitis in the computed tomography era? The American Journal of Emergency Medicine. 2009;**27**:856-858

[32] McCartan D, Fleming FJ, Grace PA. Perforated appendicitis: Does rural residency really explain the delay? Annals of Surgery. 2014;**259**:e58

[33] Kong VY, Aldous C, Clarke DL. Understanding the reasons for delay to definitive surgical care of patients with acute appendicitis in rural South Africa. South African Journal of Surgery. 2014;**52**:2-5

[34] Pande T, Mohanty Z, Nair A, et al. Seasonal variation of acute appendicitis: An armed forces experience of high altitude. Medical Journal, Armed Forces India. 2021;**77**:479-484

[35] Elliott BM, Bissett IP, Harmston C. Prehospital barriers for rural New Zealand parents in paediatric appendicitis: A qualitative analysis. ANZ Journal of Surgery. 2021;**91**:2130-2138

[36] Paquette IM, Zuckerman R, Finlayson SR. Perforated appendicitis among rural and urban patients: Implications of access to care. Annals of Surgery. 2011;**253**:534-538

[37] Edwards KH, Franklin RC, Edwards MT, Stewart RA. Requesting air ambulance transport of patients with suspected appendicitis: The decision-making process through the eyes of the rural clinician. The Australian Journal of Rural Health. 2022. DOI: 10.1111/ajr.12956

[38] Bagcchi S. Villagers in rural India stage anti-superstition march after boy dies from untreated appendicitis. BMJ. 2014;**348**:g1281

[39] Elliott BM, Witcomb Cahill H, Harmston C. Paediatric appendicitis: Increased disease severity and complication rates in rural children. ANZ Journal of Surgery. 2019;**89**:1126-1132

[40] Huang N, Yip W, Chang HJ, Chou YJ. Trends in rural and urban differentials in incidence rates for ruptured appendicitis under the National Health Insurance in Taiwan. Public Health. 2006;**120**:1055-1063

[41] Ladd MR, Pajewski NM, Becher RD, et al. Delays in treatment of pediatric appendicitis: A more accurate variable for measuring pediatric healthcare inequalities? The American Surgeon. 2013;**79**:875-881

[42] Nwomeh BC, Chisolm DJ, Caniano DA, Kelleher KJ. Racial and socioeconomic disparity in perforated appendicitis among children: Where is the problem? Pediatrics. 2006;**117**:870-875

[43] Chang YJ, Chao HC, Kong MS, et al. Misdiagnosed acute appendicitis in children in the emergency department. Chang Gung Medical Journal. 2010;**33**:551-557

[44] Jørgensen AB, Amirian I, Watt SK, et al. No circadian variation in Surgeons' ability to diagnose acute appendicitis. Journal of Surgical Education. 2016;**73**:275-280

[45] Deng Y, Chang DC, Zhang Y, et al. Seasonal and day of the week variations of perforated appendicitis in US children. Pediatric Surgery International. 2010;**26**:691-696

[46] Drake FT et al. Time-of-day and appendicitis: Impact on management and outcomes. Surgery. 2017;**161**:405-414

[47] Asad S, Ahmed A, Ahmad S, et al. Causes of delayed presentation of acute appendicitis and its impact on morbidity and mortality. Journal of Ayub Medical College, Abbottabad. 2015;**27**:620-623

[48] Castro P, Rincón J, Sánchez C, et al. Presurgical time and associated

factors as predictors of acute perforated appendicitis: A prospective cohort study in a teaching pediatric hospital in Colombia. BMC Pediatrics. 2022;**22**:49

[49] Archibong AE, Ekanem I, Jibrin P. Appendicitis in south eastern Nigerian children. The Central African Journal of Medicine. 1995;**41**:94-97

[50] Frei SP, Bond WF, Bazuro RK, et al. Is early analgesia associated with delayed treatment of appendicitis? The American Journal of Emergency Medicine. 2008;**26**:176-180

[51] Özkurt E. Factors affecting patient outcomes in acute appendicitis in rural areas: An observational cohort study. World Journal of Surgery. 2021;**45**:2337-2346

[52] Simmering JE, Polgreen LA, Talan DA, et al. Association of Appendicitis Incidence with Warmer Weather Independent of season. JAMA Network Open. 2022;**5**:e2234269

[53] Deng CY, Huang N, Chou YJ, et al. Comparison of perforation risk among physicians, other medical professionals and general adults with acute appendicitis in Taiwan. The British Journal of Surgery. 2006;**93**:1297-1302

[54] Putnam LR, Tsao K, Nguyen HT, et al. The impact of socioeconomic status on Appendiceal perforation in pediatric appendicitis. The Journal of Pediatrics. 2016;**170**:156-60.e1

[55] Bickel A, Ganam S, Abu Shakra I, et al. Delayed diagnosis and subsequently increased severity of acute appendicitis (compatible with clinical-pathologic grounds) during the COVID-19 pandemic: An observational case-control study. BMC Gastroenterology. 2022;**22**:19

[56] Burgard M, Cherbanyk F, Nassiopoulos K, et al. An effect of the COVID-19 pandemic: Significantly more complicated appendicitis due to delayed presentation of patients! PLoS One. 2021;**16**:e0249171

[57] Gerall CD, DeFazio JR, Kahan AM, et al. Delayed presentation and sub-optimal outcomes of pediatric patients with acute appendicitis during the COVID-19 pandemic. Journal of Pediatric Surgery. 2021;**56**:905-910

[58] Gaitero Tristán J, Souto Romero H, et al. Acute appendicitis in children during the COVID-19 pandemic: Neither delayed diagnosis nor worse outcomes. Pediatric Emergency Care. 2021;**37**:185-190

[59] Lin HR, Wang HC, Wang JH, Lu HH. Increased risk of perforated appendicitis in patients with schizophrenia and dementia: A population-based case-control study. Medicine (Baltimore). 2020;**99**:e18919

[60] Hung SK, Kou HW, Wu KH, et al. Does medical disparity exist while treating severe mental illness patients with acute appendicitis in emergency departments? A real-world database study. BMC Psychiatry. 2022;**22**:488

[61] Tsai SH, Hsu CW, Chen SC, et al. Complicated acute appendicitis in diabetic patients. American Journal of Surgery. 2008;**196**:34-39

[62] Timmerman ME, Groen H, Heineman E, Broens PM. The influence of underweight and obesity on the diagnosis and treatment of appendicitis in children. International Journal of Colorectal Disease. 2016;**31**:1467-1473

[63] Chao PW, Ou SM, Chen YT, et al. Acute appendicitis in patients with end-stage renal disease. Journal of Gastrointestinal Surgery. 2012;**16**:1940-1946

[64] Cobb T. Appendicitis following blunt abdominal trauma. The American Journal of Emergency Medicine. 2017;**35**:1386.e5-1386.e6

[65] Dalpiaz A, Gandhi J, Smith NL, et al. Mimicry of appendicitis symptomatology in congenital anomalies and diseases of the genitourinary system and pregnancy. Current Urology. 2017;**9**:169-178

[66] Hwang M, Wilson K, Wendt L, et al. The great gut mimicker: A case report of MIS-C and appendicitis clinical presentation overlap in a teenage patient. BMC Pediatrics. 2021;**21**:258

[67] Ueberrueck T, Koch A, Meyer L, et al. Ninety-four appendectomies for suspected acute appendicitis during pregnancy. World Journal of Surgery. 2004;**28**:508-511

[68] Basaran A, Basaran M. Diagnosis of acute appendicitis during pregnancy: A systematic review. Obstetrical & Gynecological Survey. 2009;**64**:481-488

[69] Zachariah SK, Fenn M, Jacob K, et al. Management of acute abdomen in pregnancy: Current perspectives. International Journal of Women's Health. 2019;**11**:119-134

[70] Copson S, Nathan E. Surgery in pregnancy: Identifying factors contributing to variation and delay in diagnosis and management of appendicitis in pregnancy. The Australian & New Zealand Journal of Obstetrics & Gynaecology. 2021;**61**:500-504

[71] Bostanci SA, Şenel E. The importance of physician speciality on the diagnosis of acute appendicitis and its effect on morbidity in children. Journal of Paediatrics and Child Health. 2022;**58**:2003-2007

[72] Marzuillo P, Germani C, Krauss BS, Barbi E. Appendicitis in children less than five years old: A challenge for the general practitioner. World Journal of Clinical Pediatrics. 2015;**4**:19-24

[73] Bal A, Anil M, Nartürk M, et al. Importance of clinical decision making by experienced pediatric surgeons when children are suspected of having acute appendicitis: The reality in a high-volume pediatric emergency department. Pediatric Emergency Care. 2017;**33**:e38-e42

[74] Mahajan P, Basu T, Pai CW, et al. Factors associated with potentially missed diagnosis of appendicitis in the emergency department. JAMA Network Open. 2020;**3**:e200612

[75] Bachar I, Perry ZH, Dukhno L, et al. Diagnostic value of laparoscopy, abdominal computed tomography, and ultrasonography in acute appendicitis. Journal of Laparoendoscopic & Advanced Surgical Techniques. Part A. 2013;**23**:982-989

[76] D'Souza N, Hicks G, Beable R, et al. Magnetic resonance imaging (MRI) for diagnosis of acute appendicitis. Cochrane Database of Systematic Reviews. 2021;**12**:CD012028

[77] Grunditz T, Rydén CI, Janzon L. Does the retrocecal position influence the course of acute appendicitis. Acta Chirurgica Scandinavica. 1983;**149**:707-710

[78] Castro BA, Novillo IC, Vázquez AG, et al. Impact of the appendiceal position on the diagnosis and treatment of pediatric appendicitis. Revista Paulista Pediatria. 2019;**37**:161-165

[79] Ball WR, Privitera A. Subhepatic appendicitis: a diagnostic dilemma. BML Case Reports. 2013;**2013**:bcr2013009454

[80] Akbulut S, Ulku A, Senol A, et al. Left-sided appendicitis: Review of

95 published cases and a case report. World Journal of Gastroenterology. 2010;**16**:5598-5602

[81] Parsons C, Naqvi S, Wheeler R. Intra-thoracic appendicitis in a child with Down's syndrome. Journal of Pediatric Surgery. 2013;**48**:E29-E31

[82] Raveenthiran V. Neonatal appendicitis (part 2): A review of 24 cases with inguinoscrotal manifestation. Journal of Neonatal Surgery. 2015;**4**(2):15

[83] van Dijk ST, van Dijk AH, Dijkgraaf MG, et al. Meta-analysis of in-hospital delay before surgery as a risk factor for complications in patients with acute appendicitis. The British Journal of Surgery. 2018;**105**:933-945

[84] Ingraham AM, Cohen ME, Bilimoria KY, et al. Effect of delay to operation on outcomes in adults with acute appendicitis. Archives of Surgery. 2010;**145**:886-892

[85] Yukumi S, Ishimaru K, Suzuki H, et al. Appropriate antibiotic selection during the in-hospital waiting period for surgery for appendicitis. Journal of Anus Rectum Colon. 2022;**6**:259-263

[86] Barr D, van Heerden JA, Mucha P. The diagnostic challenge of postoperative acute appendicitis. World Journal of Surgery. 1991;**15**:526-529

[87] Banerjee A, Ratan SK, Neogi S, et al. Role of ultrasonography and inflammatory markers in predicting complicated appendicitis. Journal of Indian Association of Pediatric Surgeons. 2022;**27**:448-454

[88] Sağ S, Basar D, Yurdadoğan F, et al. Comparison of appendicitis scoring Systems in Childhood Appendicitis. Turkish Achieves Pediatrics. 2022;**57**:532-537

[89] Ghareeb WM, Emile SH, Elshobaky A. Artificial intelligence compared to Alvarado scoring system alone or combined with ultrasound criteria in the diagnosis of acute appendicitis. Journal of Gastrointestinal Surgery. 2022;**26**:655-658

[90] Shikha A, Kasem A. The development and validation of artificial intelligence pediatric appendicitis decision-tree for children 0 to 12 years old. European Journal of Pediatric Surgery. 2022. DOI: 10.1055/a-1946-0157

[91] Holcomb GW, St Peter SD. Current management of complicated appendicitis in children. European Journal of Pediatric Surgery. 2012;**22**:207-212

[92] Andersson RE. The natural history and traditional management of appendicitis revisited: Spontaneous resolution and predominance of pre-hospital perforations imply that a correct diagnosis is more important than an early diagnosis. World Journal of Surgery. 2007;**31**:86-92

[93] Scher KS, Coil JA Jr. Appendicitis: Factors that influence the frequency of perforation. Southern Medical Journal. 1980;**73**:1561-1563

[94] Howell EC, Dubina ED, Lee SL. Perforation risk in pediatric appendicitis: Assessment and management. Pediatric Health Medical Therapy. 2018;**9**:135-145

[95] Bennion RS, Thompson JE, Baron EJ, Finegold SM. Gangrenous and perforated appendicitis with peritonitis: Treatment and bacteriology. Clinical Therapeutics. 1990;**12**(Suppl. C):31-44

[96] Obinwa O, Casidy M, Flynn J. The microbiology of bacterial peritonitis due to appendicitis in children. Irish Journal of Medical Science. 2014;**183**:585-591

[97] Rather SA, Bari SU, Malik AA, Khan A. Drainage vs no drainage in secondary peritonitis with sepsis following complicated appendicitis in adults in the modern era of antibiotics. World Journal Gastrointestinal Surgery. 2013;**5**:300-305

[98] Schietroma M, Piccione F, Carlei F, et al. Peritonitis from perforated appendicitis: Stress response after laparoscopic or open treatment. The American Surgeon. 2012;**78**:582-590

[99] Evbuomwan I, Onwanyin ON. Management of peritonitis in perforated appendicitis in children. East African Medical Journal. 1994;**71**:279-281

[100] Noble TB. Paralytic ileus from peritonitis after appendicitis. American Journal of Surgery. 1952;**84**:419-428

[101] Buchanan L, Tuma F. Postoperative Ileus. StatPearls Publishing; 2022

[102] Darwazeh G, Cunningham SC, Kowdley GC. A systematic review of perforated appendicitis and Phlegmon: Interval appendectomy or wait-and-see? The American Surgeon. 2016;**82**:11-15

[103] Cheng Y, Xiong X, Lu J, et al. Early versus delayed appendicectomy for appendiceal phlegmon or abscess. Cochrane Database of Systematic Reviews. 2017;**6**:CD011670

[104] Ahmed I, Deakin D, Parsons SL. Appendix mass: Do we know how to treat it? Annals of the Royal College of Surgeons of England. 2005;**87**:191-195

[105] Akingboye AA, Mahmood F, Zaman S, et al. Early versus delayed (interval) appendicectomy for the management of appendicular abscess and phlegmon: A systematic review and meta-analysis. Langenbeck's Archives of Surgery. 2021;**406**:1341-1351

[106] Andersson RE, Petzold MG. Nonsurgical treatment of appendiceal abscess or phlegmon: A systematic review and meta-analysis. Annals of Surgery. 2007;**246**:741-748

[107] van Amstel P, Sluckin TC, van Amstel T, et al. Management of appendiceal mass and abscess in children; early appendectomy or initial non-operative treatment? A systematic review and meta-analysis. Surgical Endoscopy. 2020;**34**:5234-5249

[108] Ward TE, Mangal RK, Stead TS, Ganti L. Hepatic abscess following acute appendicitis. Cureus. 2022;**14**(7):e26867

[109] Armstrong T, Dluzewski S, Yu D. Appendicitis with direct fistulation into the liver: A forgotten cause of pyogenic liver abscess. BJR Case Reports. 2020;**6**(4):20200101

[110] Saleem MM. Scrotal abscess as a complication of perforated appendicitis: A case report and review of the literature. Cases Journal. 2008;**1**:165

[111] Naidoo S, Du Toit R, Bhyat A. Perforated appendicitis presenting as a thigh abscess: A lethal combination. South African Journal of Surgery. 2016;**54**:43

[112] Faizi FR, Farzam F. Perforated retrocecal appendicitis presenting with lung abscess-a case report. Radiology Case Reports. 2022;**17**:2754-2758

[113] Carter M, Meshkat B, El-Masry S. Epidural abscess secondary to acute appendicitis. BML Case Reports. 2014;**2014**:bcr2014207446

[114] Dekkers GH, Dejong CH, Welten RJ. Splenic abscess after appendicitis. Acta Chirurgica Belgica. 2000;**100**:34-36

[115] Corder AP. Renal abscess with gas formation secondary to acute

appendicitis. British Journal of Urology. 1987;**59**:90

[116] Kawamura YJ, Sugamata Y, Yoshino K, et al. Appendico-ileo-vesical fistula. Journal of Gastroenterology. 1998;**33**:868-871

[117] McCrystal S, Kong J, Gourlas P, et al. Appendicorectal fistula with a novel solution: First case report and review of the literature. Clinical Case Reports. 2019;**7**:1885-1889

[118] Morris-Stiff GJ, Islam KA. Appendico-colic fistula complicating appendicitis in cystic fibrosis. BML Case Reports. 2010;**2010**:bcr0220102714

[119] Singh MP, Samaiya A, Sainia TK, Saxena A. Spontaneous appendico-cutaneous fistula: An unusual presentation of retroperitoneal appendicular perforation associated with psoas abscess. Journal of Surgical Case Reports. 2016;**2016**(6):rjw112

[120] Singal R, Gupta S, Mittal A, et al. Appendico-cutaneous fistula presenting as a large wound: A rare phenomenon-brief review. Acta Medica Indonesiana. 2012;**44**:53-56

[121] Killelea BK, Arkovitz MS. Perforated appendicitis presenting as appendicoumbilical fistula. Pediatric Surgery International. 2006;**22**:286-288

[122] Takeda M, Higashi Y, Shoji T, et al. Necrotizing fasciitis caused by a primary appendicocutaneous fistula. Surgery Today. 2012;**42**:781-784

[123] Reeves JM, Ip JCY. Not just a simple appendicectomy: Abdominal actinomycosis causing phlegmonous appendicitis. ANZ Journal of Surgery. 2021;**91**:E791-E792

[124] Feng W, Du XB, Zhao XF, et al. Risk factors of postoperative adhesive bowel obstruction in children with complicated appendicitis. Pediatric Surgery International. 2021;**37**:745-754

[125] Makama JG, Kache SA, Ajah LJ, Ameh EA. Intestinal obstruction caused by appendicitis: A systematic review. Journal of West African College of Surgens. 2017;**7**:94-115

[126] Casas MA, Dreifuss NH, Schlottmann F. High-volume center analysis and systematic review of stump appendicitis: Solving the pending issue. European Journal of Trauma and Emergency Surgery. 2022;**48**:1663-1672

[127] Pahari S, Shrestha M, Basukala S, et al. Complicated pylephlebitis secondary to perforated appendicitis in a child- a rare case report. Annals of Medicine Surgery (Lond). 2022;**82**:104744

[128] Bom WJ, Bolmers MD, Gans SL, et al. Discriminating complicated from uncomplicated appendicitis by ultrasound imaging, computed tomography or magnetic resonance imaging: Systematic review and meta-analysis of diagnostic accuracy. BJS Open. 2021;**5**:zraa030

[129] Kim HY, Park JH, Lee YJ, et al. Systematic review and meta-analysis of CT features for differentiating complicated and uncomplicated appendicitis. Radiology. 2018;**287**:104-115

[130] Bailey H. The Ochsner-Sherren (delayed) treatment of acute appendicitis: Indications and technique. British Medical Journal. 1930;**1**(3603):140-143

[131] Turhan AN, Kapan S, Kütükçü E, et al. Comparison of operative and non operative management of acute appendicitis. Ulusal Travma ve Acil Cerrahi Dergisi. 2009;**15**:459-462

[132] Ho CM, Chen Y, Lai HS, et al. Comparison of critical conservative treatment versus emergency operation in children with ruptured appendicitis with tumor formation. Journal of the Formosan Medical Association. 2004;**103**:359-363

[133] Simillis C, Symeonides P, Shorthouse AJ, Tekkis PP. A meta-analysis comparing conservative treatment versus acute appendectomy for complicated appendicitis (abscess or phlegmon). Surgery. 2010;**147**:818-829

[134] Cunnigaiper ND, Raj P, Ganeshram P, Venkatesan V. Does Ochsner-Sherren regimen still hold true in the management of appendicular mass? Ulusal Travma ve Acil Cerrahi Dergisi. 2010;**16**:43-46

[135] Ansaloni L, Catena F, Coccolini F, et al. Surgery versus conservative antibiotic treatment in acute appendicitis: A systematic review and meta-analysis of randomized controlled trials. Digestive Surgery. 2011;**28**:210-221

[136] Grossi U, Gallo G, Ortenzi M, et al. Changes in hospital admissions and complications of acute appendicitis during the COVID-19 pandemic: A systematic review and meta-analysis. Health Sciences Review (Oxf). 2022;**3**:100021

[137] Köhler F, Müller S, Hendricks A, et al. Changes in appendicitis treatment during the COVID-19 pandemic - a systematic review and meta-analysis. International Journal of Surgery. 2021;**95**:106148

[138] Bakker OJ. Should conservative treatment of appendicitis be first line? BMJ. 2012;**344**:e2546

[139] Tan APP, Yap TL, Cheong YL, et al. Conservative antibiotic treatment of pediatric acute uncomplicated appendicitis during the COVID-19 pandemic: A prospective comparative cohort study. Pediatric Surgery International. 2022;**39**:60

[140] Shay S, Kupietzky A, Weiss DJ, et al. Composite criteria for non-operative Management of Acute non-Complicated Appendicitis Result in low failure rates. World Journal of Surgery. 2022;**46**:69-75

[141] Tekin A, Kurtoğlu HC, Can I, Oztan S. Routine interval appendectomy is unnecessary after conservative treatment of appendiceal mass. Colorectal Disease. 2008;**10**:465-468

[142] Meshikhes AW. Appendiceal mass: Is interval appendicectomy "something of the past"? World Journal of Gastroenterology. 2011;**17**:2977-2980

[143] Sakorafas GH, Mastoraki A, Lappas C, et al. Conservative treatment of acute appendicitis: Heresy or an effective and acceptable alternative to surgery? European Journal of Gastroenterology & Hepatology. 2011;**23**:121-127

[144] Dixon MR, Haukoos JS, Park IU, Oliak D, Kumar RR, Arnell TD, et al. An assessment of the severity of recurrent appendicitis. American Journal of Surgery. 2003;**186**:718-722

[145] Raveenthiran V, Bharadwaj RA. Mucosa-coring salvage (MU-CO-SAL) Appendicectomy: A useful technique in the Management of Neglected Appendicular Mass. Journal of Indian Association of Pediatric Surgeons. 2020;**25**:239-241

[146] Neogi S, Banerjee A, Panda SS, Ratan SK, Narang R. Laparoscopic versus open appendicectomy for complicated appendicitis in children: A systematic review and meta-analysis. Journal of

Pediatric Surgery. 2022 Mar;**57**(3):394-405. DOI: 10.1016/j.jpedsurg.2021.07.005

[147] Athanasiou C, Lockwood S, Markides GA. Systematic review and meta-analysis of laparoscopic versus open Appendicectomy in adults with complicated appendicitis: An update of the literature. World Journal of Surgery. 2017;**41**(12):3083-3099. DOI: 10.1007/s00268-017-4123-3

[148] Zhang S, Du T, Jiang X, Song C. Laparoscopic appendectomy in children with perforated appendicitis: A meta-analysis. Surgical Laparoscopy, Endoscopy & Percutaneous Techniques. 2017 Aug;**27**(4):262-266. DOI: 10.1097/SLE.0000000000000411

[149] Wysocki AP, Allen J, Rey-Conde T, North JB. Mortality from acute appendicitis is associated with complex disease and co-morbidity. ANZ Journal of Surgery. 2015;**85**:521-524

[150] Goldacre MJ, Duncan ME, Griffith M, et al. Trends in mortality from appendicitis and from gallstone disease in English populations, 1979-2006: Study of multiple-cause coding of deaths. Postgraduate Medical Journal. 2011;**87**:245-250

[151] Williams BM, Purcell LN, Varela C, et al. Appendicitis mortality in a resource-limited setting: Issues of access and failure to rescue. The Journal of Surgical Research. 2021;**259**:320-325

[152] Dongarwar D, Taylor J, Ajewole V, et al. Trends in appendicitis among pregnant women, the risk for cardiac arrest, and maternal-fetal mortality. World Journal of Surgery. 2020;**44**:3999-4005

[153] Vissers RJ, Lennarz WB. Pitfalls in appendicitis. Emergency Medicine Clinics of North America. 2010;**28**:103-118

[154] Sosner E, Patlas MN, Chernyak V, et al. Missed acute appendicitis on multidetector computed tomography and magnetic resonance imaging: Legal ramifications, challenges, and avoidance strategies. Current Problems in Diagnostic Radiology. 2017;**46**:360-364

[155] Karpelowsky JS, Bickler S, Rode H. Appendicitis--pitfalls and medicolegal implications. South African Medical Journal. 2006;**96**:866-872

Chapter 4

Ultrasound Imaging of Appendicitis

Emmanuel Abiola Babington

Abstract

Ultrasound is a handy tool in diagnosing appendicitis and its possible complications. The sensitivity and specificity of ultrasound in diagnosing appendicitis can be comparable to CT and MRI owing to a highly skilled and experienced operator, high-quality equipment, and slim patients. A multi-imaging approach is advisable when ultrasound findings are inconclusive, that is, when you do not visualise the normal appendix in patients with a high clinical suspicion of appendicitis. During the ultrasound evaluation of appendicitis, it is essential to initially examine the organs of the abdomen and pelvis to rule out other mimicking pathologies before switching to a high-frequency transducer to examine the bowel and appendix. The normal appendix on ultrasound appears blind-ending, tubular, compressible, and non-peristaltic, adjacent to the caecum and terminal ileum, usually in the right iliac fossa. Adopting various ultrasound scanning techniques, including 'mowing the lawn,' 'graded compression,' and a combination of supine and lateral decubitus scanning positions, helps to improve the visualisation of the appendix and the diagnosis of appendicitis. It is imperative to differentiate between uncomplicated and complicated appendicitis by evaluating their ultrasound features. However, in some cases, there is limited imaging accuracy in making this differentiation.

Keywords: appendicolith, appendix ultrasound, bowel ultrasound, complicated appendicitis, gangrenous appendicitis, perforated appendicitis, uncomplicated appendicitis

1. Introduction

Appendicitis is the inflammation of the vermiform appendix [1]. An appropriate diagnosis remains challenging for many clinicians and imaging specialists despite being a well-known disease and a common reason for emergency operation (appendectomy) [1]. The overall clinical aim to keep the rate of negative appendectomies to the possible minimum necessitates the correct preoperative imaging diagnosis of appendicitis [2, 3]. For instance, one study [4] found a link between patients who had appendectomy and tonsillectomy in childhood having a higher risk of developing myocardial infarction later in life. While the relationship has not yet been well-established in the literature [4], this, in conjunction with surgical risks, further highlights the importance of a limited negative appendectomy rate in practice, thereby increasing the requirement of an accurate diagnosis of appendicitis clinically and on imaging.

The gold standard in the imaging of appendicitis is Computed Tomography (CT), with a sensitivity and specificity of 81–94% and 90–94%, respectively, and readily available to many emergency departments in the western world [5]. Furthermore, Magnetic Resonance Imaging (MRI), with a sensitivity and specificity of 96%, respectively, is very useful in diagnosing appendicitis, particularly in pregnant women [5]. However, there is a growing interest in using Ultrasound (US) as the first line of appendicitis imaging, with a conditional CT scan when US findings are equivocal [5–7].

Unlike CT and MRI, US has a varying but lower sensitivity of 35% - 90% and a specificity of up to 90%; however, it uses high-frequency sound waves, which are primarily known to remain harmless within diagnostic frequencies [8]. On the other hand, CT uses ionising radiation that poses some risks, particularly to children and women of childbearing age, and is potentially more expensive than US [8]. For instance, one study [9] revealed the presence of a link between patients with cancer and previous exposure to CT radiation, with CT abdomen and pelvis being one of the culprits; therefore highlighting the importance of avoiding unnecessary radiation to our patients and reinforcing the need for US as the first line of imaging in appendicitis. MRI, though relatively safe, is not cheap and may sometimes require sedation in children to keep still for the examination, which is not always practical in real-life situations [10]. MRI also has less accessibility when compared to US [10]. However, there are some drawbacks with ultrasound in examining for appendicitis which include; difficulty in scanning patients with high BMI, a high degree of transducer tenderness leading to limited visualisation of the structures, and the most significant limitation is that US is highly operator dependent, hence the variability in its sensitivity [11]. Some main factors that improve the diagnostic accuracy of US in appendicitis include; a highly skilled operator, good quality ultrasound equipment, and patient characteristics.

This chapter aims to provide some information on the ultrasound anatomy and appearances of the normal appendix, uncomplicated appendicitis, and complicated appendicitis, i.e., gangrenous and perforated appendicitis, and to provide some information on how to acquire the US images, and how to recognise different US patterns encountered in practice. These are achieved by extracting useful information from a combination of the current and relevant literature on this topic, a reflection on the author's many years of experience in carrying out ultrasound examinations of appendicitis, and the knowledge obtained from numerous training sessions delivered by other experts from across the globe.

2. Training and quality control

Globally, US evaluation of appendicitis is generally performed daily across diverse professional specialties in the hospital, ranging from sonographers, radiologists, emergency physicians, gastroenterologists, and general practitioners. Therefore, this chapter will collectively refer to these as 'the ultrasound examiner.'

The need for appropriate training in the area cannot be overemphasised for an accurate understanding of the various imaging appearances of an inflamed appendix and a correct diagnosis of appendicitis. In addition, it is imperative to understand the basic anatomy of the appendix, its usual location, orientation, and relationship to the neighbouring bowel anatomically and pathologically. The latter will be discussed later in this chapter. Also, it is advisable to follow up on the outcomes of cases examined and to welcome feedback from referring clinicians and surgeons, which helps with better development.

Furthermore, understanding the US machine's knobology, transducer selection, and fundamental ultrasound physics, among others, will help the ultrasound examiner with the safe and efficient usage of the US equipment to maximise its diagnostic potential. Although details of the latter are beyond the scope of this chapter, the next section will provide some relevant information regarding the US equipment.

3. Equipment

There are different kinds of US machines ranging from whole units to portables; tabletop and handheld machines with wireless display connectivity to regular mobile devices and tablets for ease of use within the hospital and community setting [12]. An appropriate US examination in the evaluation of appendicitis requires a combination of a curved-array transducer with a frequency range of 1–6.5 MHz (C1–6), a 'medium range' high-frequency linear-array transducer of 9 MHz (9 L), and occasionally, a higher frequency linear-array transducer of up to 15 MHz (15 L) for examining the appendix in younger children, and very slim adults [13]. However, in practice, the 9 L transducer is usually sufficient in evaluating the appendix in most patients after using the C1–6 in examining the other abdomen and pelvic organs for pathologies that might mimic appendicitis; like cholelithiasis, gynaecological and renal pathologies.

4. Ultrasound terminologies and scanning techniques

4.1 Terminologies and pattern recognition

For clarity to those new to ultrasound; the primary term used to describe structures/patterns displayed on US imaging is called 'echogenicity' or 'echotexture,' which is based on the level of interaction between the ultrasound beams and the individual tissue, i.e., anatomical or pathological structure seen within the region being insonated. For instance, because clear fluid allows a 'through transmission' of the ultrasound beam, this is therefore represented on the display monitor as 'anechogenic' or 'anechoic' with an increased posterior acoustic enhancement. On the other hand, structures with a high calcium content, e.g., bones and other calcifications like appendicoliths, reflect most of the ultrasound beam to the transducer, therefore appearing 'hyperechogenic' or 'hyperechoic' with posterior acoustic shadowing. Other structures between the spectrum mentioned above, like pus, masses, and purulent appendiceal contents, are sometimes described as 'hypoechoic' with reference to the surrounding anatomical structures, depending on their content.

4.2 Doppler ultrasound

Doppler Imaging, i.e., Colour (CD) and Power Doppler (PD), are mandatory functions used during US examination of appendicitis to check for evidence of vascularity which has been directly linked to inflammatory activities evident mostly in uncomplicated appendicitis [14]. While CD function is usually sufficient on most newer US equipment to interrogate for vascularity within and around the inflamed appendix, PD is also sometimes beneficial in evaluating traces of vascularity with limited detectability on CD [14]. The application of these functionalities and the adoption of appropriate scanning techniques will improve and maximise the diagnostic efficacy of ultrasound in appendicitis. The ultrasound examiner must optimise the US machine's CD setting during the evaluation of appendicitis; this is done by ensuring that the Pulse Repetition Frequency (PRF) or 'scale' is adjusted to help detect slow blood flow velocities within the region [15]. If the PRF is set too high, 'aliasing' may occur, leading to a false negative diagnosis of hypervascularity [15]. Furthermore, most US machines have other functions like Microvascular Imaging (MI) or superb microvascular imaging (SMI) and B Flow Imaging (B Flow) that are designed to have more sensitivity than CD [16, 17]. However, their nomenclatures may vary across manufacturers.

4.3 Scanning technique

The common symptoms of appendicitis include the acute onset of periumbilical or central abdominal pain, eventually radiating to the right iliac fossa (RIF) [18]. This abdominal pain can sometimes be vague, particularly in children, and can mimic symptoms of some other abdominal or gynaecological pathologies [18]. Therefore, it is highly recommended that an ultrasound examination of appendicitis should initially include; the entire abdomen and pelvis to rule out pathologies that might mimic appendicitis, and the rest of the bowel, before becoming more focused on the appendix in the RIF [19]. The patient is initially examined in a supine position, then asked to turn to the left lateral decubitus position to aid a better visualisation of the appendix.

4.3.1 Mowing the lawn

A curvilinear transducer with a frequency range of 2–6.5 MHz should be initially used in examining the abdomen and pelvic organs to rule out common pathologies like cholelithiasis, nephrolithiasis, possible signs of pyelonephritis, ovarian cysts, among others. Furthermore, using the same transducer, the examiner should continue by imaging the bowel from the LIF in the region of the sigmoid colon (usually in a fixed location) in a 'lawn-mowing' fashion to the RIF to rule out some bowel pathologies like inflammatory bowel diseases (IBD), diverticulitis, ileocecitis, and the like [19]. During the examination, a gentle and slow movement of the high-frequency transducer in a vertical sweeping direction across the abdomen helps examine most parts of the small and large bowel [19].

4.3.2 Graded compression

Subsequently, the examiner should switch to a 9 MHz linear transducer to reexamine the bowel again (as described in Section 5.3.1.); slowly from the LIF to the RIF with the final focus on the site of the patient's pain (expectedly the RIF) while applying graded compression on the abdomen throughout the examination. Graded compression, first described in 1986 by JB Puyleart [20], is an essential aspect of ultrasound imaging in appendicitis. It is described as the use of the (linear) transducer to apply gentle and gradual yet firm pressure on the abdomen to displace the bowel gas and luminal content, bringing the examined bowel structure (and pathology) closer to the view of the ultrasound transducer and the examiner [20].

4.4 Other ultrasound techniques

A transvaginal examination can be offered to some female patients when the inflamed appendix extends into the right hemipelvis or when there is a gynaecological pathology that is not well visualised on the transabdominal US imaging [21]. However, adequate prior training and competence are advised before undergoing such an intimate examination.

There is a growing increase in the roles of newer ultrasound techniques like contrast-enhanced ultrasound (CEUS) and elastography in diagnosing appendicitis. However, these are not yet well established across literature and require conventional ultrasound expertise to be performed correctly, and also not routinely used in the diagnostic workup and classification of appendicitis [22–24]. Ultimately, it is crucial to work in line with the hospital/imaging department's protocols and to work based on individual patients' requirements while respecting the patient's dignity and privacy throughout the examination.

5. Ultrasound anatomy

The normal appendix measures between 2 cm - 10 cm in length and ≤ 0.6 cm in anteroposterior (AP) dimension, having its base attached to the inferior surface of the caecum in the RIF, and its body and fundal tip in varying orientation, depending on; the location of the caecum, the length of the appendix, and its orientation of attachment to the caecum [25]. The appendix is predominantly antecaecal in orientation; however, some are retrocaecal, pelvic, and in rare cases, subhepatic, with the base usually only a few centimetres distal to the ileocaecal junction [25, 26]. On US, the normal appendix (**Figure 1**) appears as a blind-ending, tubular, compressible, and non-peristaltic loop of bowel with its base adjoining the distal end of the caecum and in a slightly inferior position to the terminal ileum and ileocaecal junction [25, 26]. It is

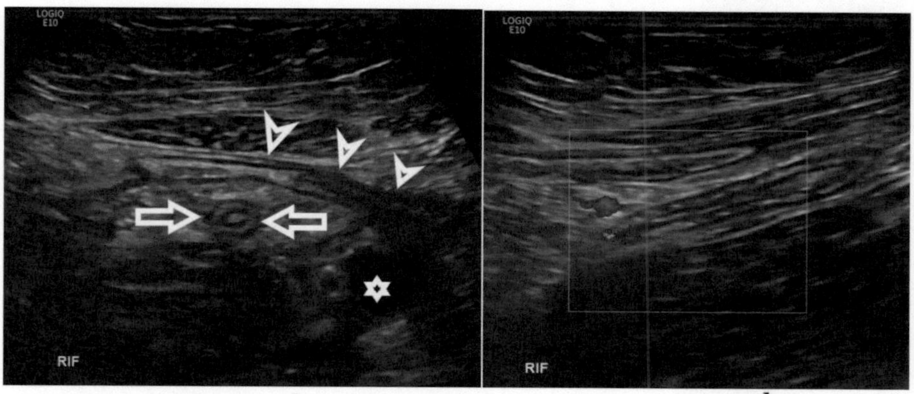

a. b.

Figure 1.
Sonograms of the normal appendix from the same patient. A: The normal appendix (between arrows) in a transverse orientation; note the 'target' appearance and the longitudinal segment of the terminal ileum (TI) coursing anterior to the appendix (arrow heads), and the iliac artery (star). b: The longitudinal segment of the appendix in a longitudinal orientation, with no appreciable flow seen on colour Doppler; also note the terminal ileum in an oblique orientation anterior to the appendix and the psoas posteriorly.

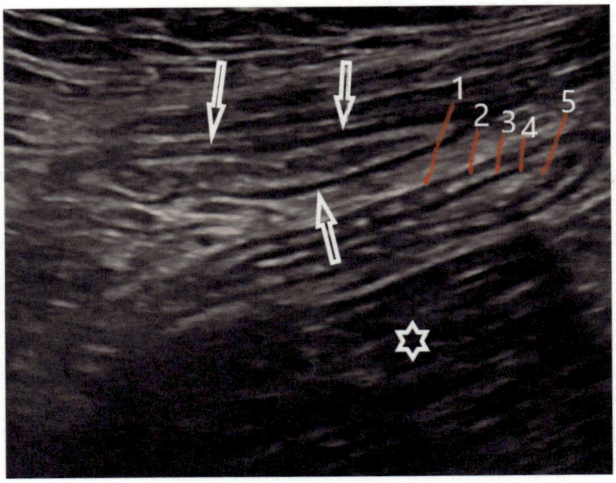

Figure 2.
Sonogram of the normal appendix in a longitudinal orientation showing its individual wall layers (numbered 1–5), with the obliquely imaged terminal ileum (between arrows) anterior to the appendix and the psoas (star) muscle.

also commonly inferior-medial to the right psoas muscle and the right external iliac vessels (**Figures 1** and **2**). In rare cases, the appendix can be seen extending into the right hemipelvis or slightly higher in an ascending fashion towards the subhepatic region [25, 26].

Like the rest of the bowel, on ultrasound, the normal appendix; usually with barely any flow evidence on CD (**Figure 1b**), has five concentric layers [27] of hyper-hypoechogenicity (see **Figure 2**), namely:

1. Hyperechoic serosa (outermost layer)

2. Hypoechoic muscularis propria

3. Hyperechoic submucosa

4. Hypoechoic mucosa

5. Hyperechoic mucosal interface (innermost/luminal layer)

However, routinely on ultrasound, only three of these five layers are easily visualised in a normal appendix: the mucosa, mucosal interface, and submucosa, with the latter being the most apparent echogenic layer [27]. In practice, care must be taken by the ultrasound examiner when measuring the appendix not to confuse the submucosal layer for the outermost serosa, as this is a habitual error made by beginners which can lead to an under-measurement of the appendix and consequently a false negative diagnosis, further delaying patient's management. Owing to this, always measure the appendix (**Figure 3a**) from serosa to serosa (S2S) to cover its maximum outer diameter (MOD). Therefore, visualising and identifying the individual layer of the appendix is essential in the proper diagnosis of (uncomplicated) appendicitis on ultrasound [28].

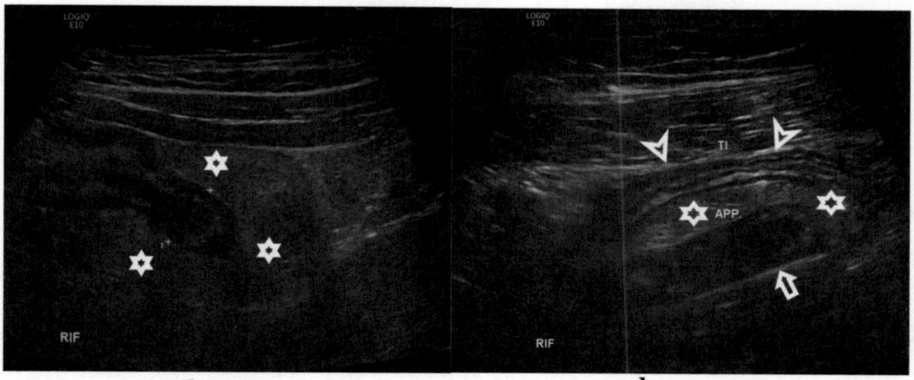

Figure 3.
Uncomplicated appendicitis sonograms acquired from different patients. A: Shows the inflamed appendix (between callipers) measuring 10 mm (MOD) from serosa to serosa (S2S), also note the echogenic periappendiceal mesenteric fat wrapping/mesenteric oedema (stars) around the inflamed appendix. b: Shows an inflamed appendix (APP., arrow) in a longitudinal orientation with mild periappendiceal mesenteric oedema (stars) and normal terminal ileum (TI, arrow heads) seen coursing anterior to the appendix from the distal ileum towards the caecum in the RIF (not imaged).

6. Uncomplicated appendicitis

6.1 Overview

Uncomplicated appendicitis is the inflammation of the appendix without any further complications [29]. It is now believed that uncomplicated and complicated appendicitis are of two separate entities and etiologies; therefore, one does not lead to the other [30]. Although details of the causes and treatment options of uncomplicated and complicated appendicitis are beyond the scope of this chapter, features seen on ultrasound to help in the correct diagnosis of uncomplicated appendicitis are discussed in the subsections below.

6.2 Ultrasound features

An inflamed appendix on ultrasound appears as a blind-ending, tubular, non-compressible, and non-peristaltic bowel structure, usually in the RIF measuring >0.6 cm in AP dimension from S2S [31].

The primary ultrasound features of uncomplicated appendicitis [31, 32] include (**Figure 3**);

- Visualisation of an inflamed non-compressible appendix measuring above 0.6 cm,
- Increased echogenicity of the periappendiceal mesentery (i.e., mesenteric oedema) and
- The visualised appendix corresponding to the site of the patient's maximum transducer tenderness.

In addition, the secondary ultrasound features [28, 33] of uncomplicated appendicitis are;

- Mesenteric lymphadenopathy,
- Increased appendiceal wall vascularity (**Figure 4**),
- Moderate amount of free fluid in the RIF, and
- Free fluid in other regions of the abdomen and pelvis.

To further emphasise; in order to rule out appendicitis on ultrasound, the normal appendix (see Section 6) must be visualised [34]. In the absence of the latter, the ultrasound report should generally be along the lines of '*the appendix has not been visualised; however, no secondary ultrasound features of appendicitis seen.*' Owing to the expectation that the examination was correctly done using the proper scanning techniques, equipment, and that the US examiner has accomplished appropriate US training (explained in the previous sections).

6.3 Hypervascularity

Ultrasound reveals hypervascularity of an inflamed appendix as the increase in colour Doppler flow (CDF) signal within the wall of the appendix (**Figure 4**); most commonly the echogenic submucosa layer (**Figure 3b**), which is also the most prominent layer seen on US in uncomplicated appendicitis [35]. Usually, the presence of CDF within the walls of an inflamed appendix without any features of complications (Section 9) confirms the diagnosis of uncomplicated appendicitis and potentially rules out a gangrenous appendix [35].

6.4 Focal appendicitis

Focal appendicitis occurs when only a region of the appendix is inflamed (**Figure 5**), affecting mainly the appendix base or fundal region; this can lead to a false

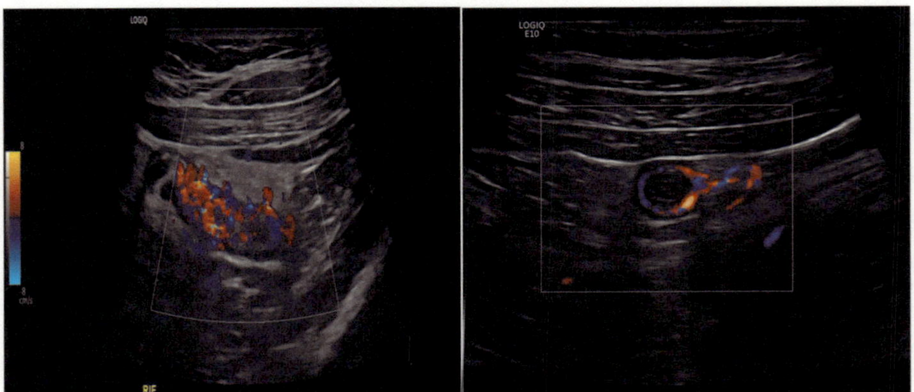

a. b.

Figure 4.
*Sonograms acquired from different patients showing hypervascularity in uncomplicated appendicitis. A: Shows an inflamed appendix in a longitudinal orientation with significantly increased vascularity affecting roughly all the layers of the appendix; note the low PRF setting on the colour scale to the left of the image. b: Shows a transverse cross-section of the fundus of a focally inflamed appendix; note that the increased vascularity seen affects only the submucosa layer of the wall of the appendix (same patient as in **Figure 5**).*

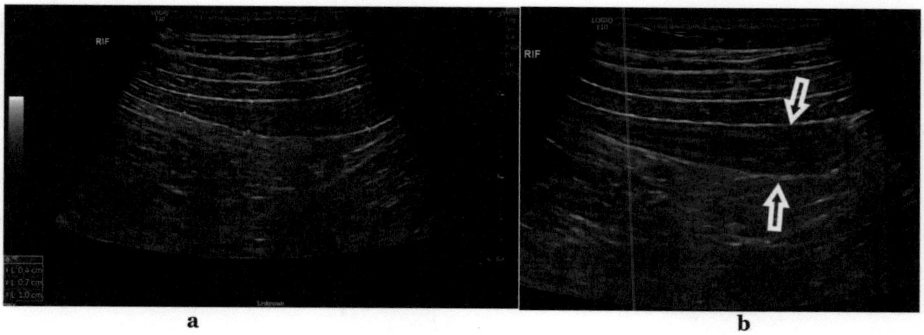

Figure 5.
Sonograms obtained from the same patient showing focal appendicitis that mainly affected the fundal region of the appendix. A: Shows the appendix with callipers measuring varying sections from S2S; the base measured 0.4 cm, the body 0.7 cm, and the fundal tip measured 1.0 cm in AP calibres. b: Shows the blind end of the focally inflamed appendix (between arrows) with no significant periappendiceal mesenteric oedema.

negative ultrasound diagnosis if the appendix has not been examined in its entirety [33, 36]. This highlights the importance of visualising all parts of the appendix during an US examination. Therefore, it is mandatory to state in the ultrasound report the study limitations encountered if a complete diagnosis was not attained, availing the patient of prompt diagnosis by another ultrasound examiner or other imaging modalities.

6.5 Atypical uncomplicated appendicitis

Some atypical cases of appendicitis occasionally diagnosed on ultrasound include; long (or high) ascending retrocecal appendicitis (LARA), pelvic appendicitis (PA) using the transabdominal and possibly transvaginal approach, and appendicitis during pregnancy (ADP).

6.5.1 Appendicitis during pregnancy (ADP)

The sensitivity of US in the detection of ADP is known to be low, and it further declines as the pregnancy progresses; for instance, one study [37] found a sensitivity of 69%, 63%, and 51% in the first, second, and third trimesters respectively. Their respective specificity was 85%, 85%, and 65% [37]. During pregnancy, the appendix and the rest of the bowel 'give way' to the growing gravid uterus; therefore, personnel experience plays a crucial role in visualising the appendix with ultrasound in these patients, as the appendix will tend to be located higher or in a more lateral position than in a non-pregnant patient [37, 38]. Owing to this, MRI, with much higher sensitivity and specificity than US, is considered the imaging modality of choice in this case if ultrasound is inconclusive or unavailable [38].

6.5.2 Pelvic appendicitis (PA)

PA occurs when an inflamed appendix extends into the pelvis (majorly the right hemipelvis), with an US appearance of a blind-ending, tubular, non-peristaltic bowel loop medial (**Figure 6a**) or lateral (**Figure 6b**) to the right ovary measuring >0.6 cm with evidence of hypervascularity (**Figure 6c**), which in some cases will present with

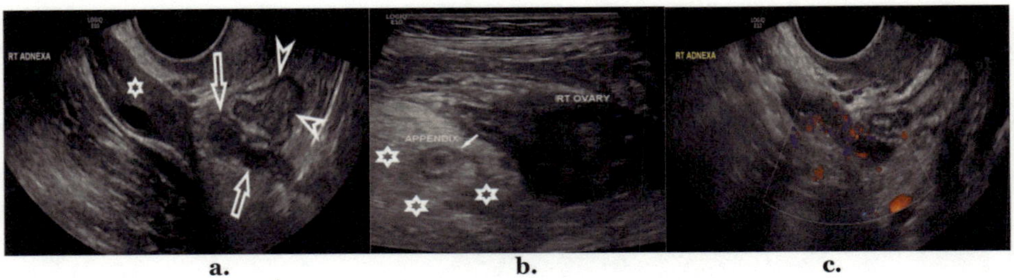

Figure 6.
Pelvic appendicitis. A: A transvaginal sonogram of the right hemipelvis showing the right ovary (star), an inflamed appendix (arrows), and a slightly thick-walled adjacent bowel loop (arrow heads) secondary to the inflamed appendix. b: A transabdominal sonogram of the right hemipelvis obtained using a 9 MHz linear transducer with the appendix (arrow) and some echogenic periappendiceal mesenteric oedema (stars), and the normal right ovary medial to it. c: Shows hypervascularity on colour Doppler of the inflamed appendix of the same patient in a.

increased adjacent bowel wall thickening secondary to the inflamed appendix (**Figure 6a**) [21]. The inflamed appendix usually corresponds to the site of the patient's maximum tenderness and elicits a pain response when in contact with the ultrasound transducer [21].

6.5.3 Long ascending retrocecal appendicitis (LARA)

In the case of LARA, the inflamed appendix courses craniomedial to the psoas muscle (**Figure 7**) from its basal connection to the caecum in the RIF towards the subhepatic region (Video 1, https://youtu.be/BhE1OIzoKLI), and due to its location, patients with LARA can present with symptoms mimicking other abdominal pathologies like biliary or urinary pathologies [39]. Therefore, a thorough examination of the other abdominal organs and a careful identification of the other bowel structures like the terminal ileum and caecum can help the ultrasound examiner to locate the appendix in this case.

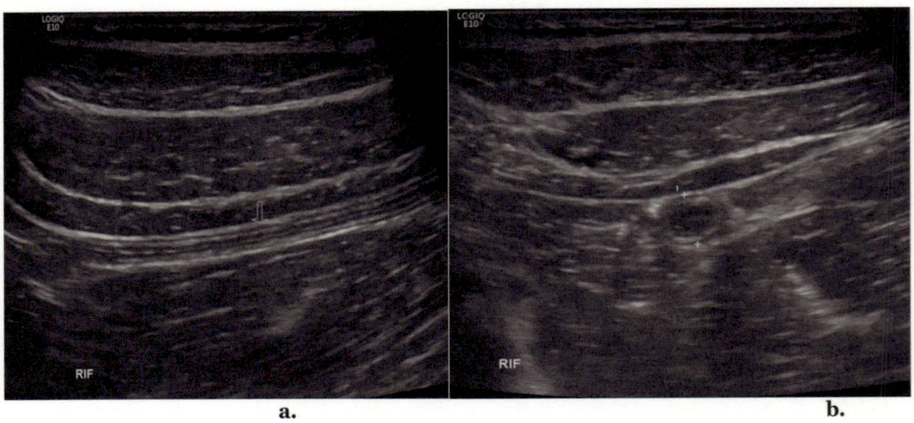

Figure 7.
Long ascending retrocecal appendix. (a) Reveals a sonogram acquired with the patient in a left lateral decubitus position, showing a long retrocecal appendix (arrow) coursing medial to the psoas muscle (posterior surface) and extending towards the right subhepatic region. The appendix was focally inflamed at the base, as seen in (b), where it measured 0.7 cm (between callipers), while the rest of the appendix appeared normal. ***Video 1*** *(https://youtu.be/BhE1OIzoKLI) shows the long ascending retrocecal appendix in transverse orientation with some reactive lymph nodes seen adjacent.*

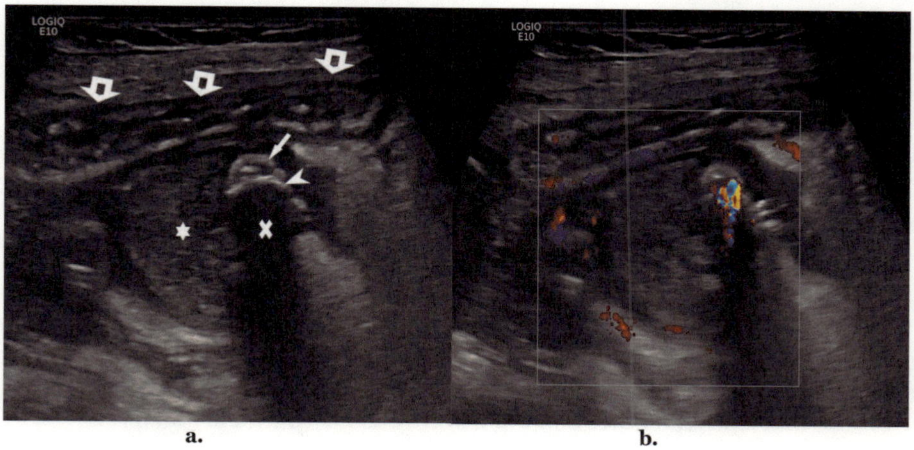

Figure 8.
An appendicolith in a patient with complicated (perforated) appendicitis. A: Shows a transverse sonogram of the appendix base (long arrow) with an appendicolith (arrow head) showing a 'strong' posterior acoustic shadow (x), periappendiceal mesenteric oedema, complex periappendiceal collection (star), and mild wall thickening of the adjacent terminal ileum (three short arrows) anteriorly. b: Shows the colour Doppler mode in the same patient with a 'twinkling artefact' seen emanating from the appendicolith and mild wall hypervascularity of the terminal ileum secondary to the inflamed appendix. The ultrasound diagnosis was complicated appendicitis with possible perforation, confirmed in surgery and histopathology the next day.

7. Appendicoliths

Appendicoliths are calcified structures seen within the lumen of the appendix [40]. They are formed from an aggregation of faecal materials that calcifies over time and are usually made up of calcium phosphatase with some faecal and organic matter [40]. Known as a common culprit in the occlusion of the appendiceal lumen leading to appendicitis, however, appendicoliths have been found in many patients without appendicitis [41]. On US, appendicoliths appear as an echogenic (calcific) structure seen within the lumen of the appendix and usually present with posterior acoustic shadowing caused by a near-complete reflection of the US beam on it (**Figure 8**) [42]. The presence of an appendicolith in an inflamed appendix will usually warrant appendectomy, as appendicoliths have been known to cause a significant failure rate of non-operative management of appendicitis, which is due to the bacteria in the appendicolith forming a nidus [43]. Furthermore, an appendicolith within an inflamed appendix can traverse its wall, leading to perforation and other significant complications [44]. More information on appendicolith can be found in this recent narrative review [44].

8. Complicated (gangrenous and perforated) appendicitis

8.1 Overview

Complicated appendicitis mainly comprises gangrenous and perforated appendicitis with appendiceal necrosis [45]. These are known to lead to failed antibiotics management; therefore, surgery is always required, which can be either laparoscopic or open appendectomy, depending on the degree of complication [45–47]. In light of this, imaging plays a vital role in their differentiation [47]. Although there is a low sensitivity of imaging, recorded in literature, in distinguishing between uncomplicated and complicated appendicitis; with US even lower than CT, recognising the standard US features can make a difference in the patient's diagnostic journey while averting unnecessary radiation exposure, particularly in children and young adults [48].

8.2 Ultrasound features

The primary US features [46] of complicated appendicitis (**Figure 9**) include;

- An inflamed appendix measuring above 0.6 cm (usually above 1.0 cm) in AP calibre that can sometimes contain heterogeneous (purulent) materials
- A loss of appendiceal wall stratification, particularly loss of the submucosal layer
- The absence of wall vascularity
- The presence of an appendicolith (usually large in size)
- The visualisation of an appendiceal wall defect or mucosal ulceration and some periappendiceal fluid
- The presence of periappendiceal heterogeneous collection/abscess.

The secondary US features [46] include:

- The presence of significant mesenteric oedema

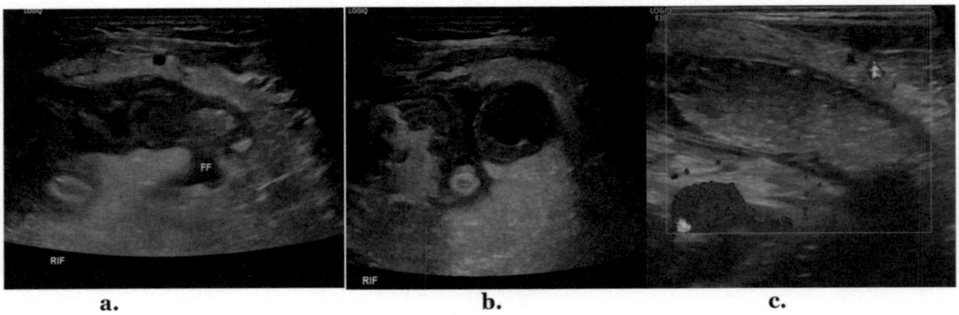

Figure 9.
Sonograms in two different patients with perforated and gangrenous appendicitis confirmed surgically and histopathologically. A: Shows a significantly inflamed appendix measuring 18 mm AP (not shown in the image) in a longitudinal orientation with an abnormal wall layering, including a loss of the echogenic submucosal layer and significant echogenic periappendiceal mesenteric oedema. Also, note the small area in the posterior surface of the appendix with tracking fluid (FF) from a likely compromised serosa, which raised the suspicion of perforated appendicitis on ultrasound. b: Shows the same appendix in transverse orientation with significant periappendiceal mesenteric oedema and an abnormal appendix wall stratification. c: Shows a longitudinal image of another patient with a gangrenous appendix filled with purulent content. This appendix is thin-walled and has lost its submucosa layer, with its lumen filled with echogenic (purulent) content. No wall or luminal vascularity was seen, although not shown in the image; this patient also had a large appendicolith at the base of the appendix that likely caused the complication.

- The presence of a sizeable unexplainable mass-like structure seen where the appendix is expected to be, without visualising the appendix

- The presence of some free fluid in the abdomen and pelvis.

In addition, tiny echogenic punctate foci within the wall of the appendix (intramural) have been associated with possible appendix necrosis and gangrene (**Figure 9c**). However, the ultrasound examiner must take care not to misidentify this sign with the bowel gas in the adjacent normal bowel structures [49]. Furthermore, the loss of the normal appendiceal wall stratification (**Figure 8a** and **b**) and the visualisation of a defect in the appendix wall or mucosal ulceration with a close relation to a collected periappendiceal fluid (**Figure 9a**) or collection (**Figure 8a**) significantly raises the suspicion of perforation on US [50, 51].

9. Other pathologies with similar symptoms

In practice, not every patient presenting with the symptoms of appendicitis ends up having appendicitis. There are many other disease conditions that are either bowel-related or extra-bowel pathologies with symptoms that mimic appendicitis in the abdomen and pelvis. Some commonly encountered bowel-related appendicitis-mimicking pathologies diagnosed on ultrasound are; Crohn's disease and ulcerative colitis (IBD), diverticulitis, caecitis, terminal ileitis, ileocecitis, colitis, mesenteric adenitis, and intussusception [52]. These all have individual identifying features on ultrasound that help distinguish the diagnosis from appendicitis; however, this is beyond the scope of this chapter.

Meanwhile, some non-bowel-related pathologies encountered on US with symptoms that mimic appendicitis are; cholelithiasis with or without cholecystitis, urinary tract infection, pyelonephritis, nephrolithiasis/urolithiasis, and gynaecological (including ovarian-related) pathologies [53]. It is the responsibility of the ultrasound examiner to identify and properly diagnose these conditions when visualised on ultrasound or determine if the appearances are inconclusive, therefore promptly suggesting other diagnostic imaging examinations to prevent unanticipated complications.

10. Summary

Ultrasound is a handy and safe tool in diagnosing appendicitis with a consistently improving diagnostic efficacy in line with technological advancement and increased availability of information. However, due to its significant operator dependence, a high degree of training and competence is required, particularly in the area of diagnosis of appendicitis. In addition, certain factors improve the sensitivity and specificity of ultrasound in examining for appendicitis; this includes the use of good scanning equipment, an understanding of the bowel ultrasound anatomy and various (typical and atypical) presentations and complications of appendicitis, and the adoption of the proper scanning techniques. This chapter discussed the scanning techniques and ultrasound appearances commonly encountered in patients with appendicitis, and it also presented some relevant sonograms of normal and abnormal appendixes that were confirmed surgically and histologically.

Acknowledgements

Many thanks L.D. Sander and Dr. Babalola Afolabi for their effort in proofreading the manuscript of this chapter.

Conflict of interest

No conflict of interest.

Author details

Emmanuel Abiola Babington
Sheffield Hallam University, University Hospitals of Leicester NHS Trust, Leicester, UK

*Address all correspondence to: emmanuel.babington@uhl-tr.nhs.uk

References

[1] Stringer MD. Acute appendicitis. Journal of Paediatrics and Child Health. 2017;**53**(11):1071-1076. DOI: 10.1111/jpc.13737

[2] Ceresoli M, Coccolini F, Magnone S, Lucianetti A, Bisagni P, Armao T, et al. The decrease of non-complicated acute appendicitis and the negative appendectomy rate during pandemic. European Journal of Trauma and Emergency Surgery. 2021;**47**(5):1359-1365. DOI: 10.1007/s00068-021-01663-7

[3] Garcia EM, Camacho MA, Karolyi DR, Kim DH, Cash BD, Chang KJ. Expert panel on gastrointestinal imaging. ACR appropriateness criteria® right lower quadrant pain-suspected appendicitis. Journal of the American College of Radiology. 2018;**15**(11S):S373-S387. DOI: 10.1016/j.jacr.2018.09.033

[4] Janszky I, Mukamal KJ, Dalman C, Hammar N, Ahnve S. Childhood appendectomy, tonsillectomy, and risk for premature acute myocardial infarction—A nationwide population-based cohort study. European Heart Journal. 2011;**32**(18):2290-2296. DOI: 10.1093/eurheartj/ehr137

[5] Bom WJ, Bolmers MD, Gans SL, van Rossem CC, van Geloven AAW, Bossuyt PMM, et al. Discriminating complicated from uncomplicated appendicitis by ultrasound imaging, computed tomography or magnetic resonance imaging: Systematic review and meta-analysis of diagnostic accuracy. BJS open. 2021;**5**(2):zraa 030. DOI: 10.1093/bjsopen/zraa030

[6] Darbyshire AR, Towers A, Harrison R, Taylor M, Carter NC, Toh SKC, et al. Routine ultrasound for suspected appendicitis in children: A single-Centre retrospective cohort study. The Annals of The Royal College of Surgeons of England. 2022;**0**:0-0. DOI: 10.1308/rcsann.2021.0326

[7] Bom WJ, Scheijmans JCG, Salminen P, Boermeester MA. Diagnosis of uncomplicated and complicated appendicitis in adults. Scandinavian Journal of Surgery. 2021;**110**(2):170-179. DOI: 10.1177/14574969211008330

[8] Eng KA, Abadeh A, Ligocki C, Lee YK, Moineddin R, Adams-Webber T, et al. Acute appendicitis: A meta-analysis of the diagnostic accuracy of US, CT, and MRI as second-line imaging tests after an initial US. Radiology. 2018;**288**(3):717-727. DOI: 10.1148/radiol.2018180318

[9] Pearce MS, Salotti JA, Little MP, McHugh K, Lee C, Kim KP, Howe NL, Ronckers CM. Sir Craft AW, Parker L, Berrington de González A. Radiation exposure from CT scans in childhood and subsequent risk of leukaemia and brain tumours: A retrospective cohort study. Lancet. 2012;**380**(9840):499-505. DOI: 10.1016/s0140-6736(12)60815-0

[10] Zisman A, Novi B, Gaughan J, Carr L. Factors affecting utilization of CT scan following ultrasound evaluation of suspected appendicitis. Journal of Osteopathic Medicine. 2022;**122**(6):313-318. DOI: 10.1515/jom-2021-0251

[11] Yuan F, Necas M. Retrospective audit of patients presenting for ultrasound with suspicion of appendicitis. Australasian Journal of Ultrasound in Medicine. 2015;**18**(2):67-69. DOI: 10.1002/j.2205-0140.2015.tb00044.x

[12] Mathur S. Recent Advancements in ultrasound machines and ultrasound imaging. 2021. Available from: https://www.primedeq.com/blog/recent-advancements-in-ultrasound-imaging/

[13] Elliott CL, Maclachlan J, Beal I. Paediatric bowel ultrasound in inflammatory bowel disease. European Journal of Radiology. 2018;**108**:21-27. DOI: 10.1016/j.ejrad.2018.09.004

[14] Petroianu A. Diagnosis of acute appendicitis. International Journal of Surgery. 2012;**10**(3):115-119. DOI: 10.1016/j.ijsu.2012.02.006

[15] Kim MS, Kwon HJ, Kang KA, Do IG, Park HJ, Kim EY, et al. Diagnostic performance and useful findings of ultrasound re-evaluation for patients with equivocal CT features of acute appendicitis. The British Journal of Radiology. 2018;**91**(1082):20170529. DOI: 10.1259/bjr.20170529

[16] Yen HH. Progress in the ultrasonographic microvascular imaging. Journal of Medical Ultrasound. 2018; **26**(1):1. DOI: 10.4103/JMU.JMU_28_18

[17] Hancerliogullari Koksalmis G. Drivers to adopting B-flow ultrasonography: Contextualizing the integrated technology acceptance model. BMC Medical Imaging. 2019;**19**(1):1-13. DOI: 10.1186/s12880-019-0356-y

[18] Demir MK, Savas Y, Furuncuoglu Y, Cevher T, Demiral S, Tabandeh B, et al. Imaging findings of the unusual presentations, associations and clinical mimics of acute appendicitis. The Eurasian Journal of Medicine. 2017; **49**(3):198. DOI: 10.5152/eurasianjmed.2017.17218

[19] Rodgers PM, Verma R. Transabdominal ultrasound for bowel evaluation. Radiologic Clinics. 2013; **51**(1):133-148. DOI: 10.1016/j.rcl.2012.09.008

[20] Puylaert JB. Acute appendicitis: US evaluation using graded compression. Radiology. 1986;**158**(2):355-360. DOI: 10.1148/radiology.158.2.2934762

[21] Shaaban AM, Rezvani M, Olpin JD, Kennedy AM, Gaballah AH, Foster BR, et al. Nongynecologic findings seen at pelvic US. Radiographics. 2017;**37**(7): 2045-2062. DOI: 10.1148/rg.2017170083

[22] Arslan H, Akdemir Z, Yavuz A, Gökçal F, Parlakgümüş C, İslamoglu N, et al. Efficacy of strain elastography in diagnosis and staging of acute appendicitis in pediatric patients. Medical Science Monitor: International Medical Journal of Experimental and Clinical Research. 2018;**24**:855. DOI: 10.12659/MSM.905927

[23] Isik IA, Ozkan MB. Evaluation of the clinical effectiveness of shear wave elastography in pediatric cases with acute appendicitis. Ultrasound Quarterly. 2021;**37**(2):173-177. DOI: 10.1097/RUQ.0000000000000556

[24] Cozzi D, Agostini S, Bertelli E, Galluzzo M, Papa E, Scevola G, et al. Contrast-enhanced ultrasound (CEUS) in non-traumatic abdominal emergencies. Ultrasound International Open. 2020;**6**(03):E76-E86. DOI: 10.1055/a-1347-5875

[25] Castro BA, Novillo IC, Vázquez AG, Garcia PY, Herrero EF, Fraile AG. Impact of the appendiceal position on the diagnosis and treatment of pediatric appendicitis. Revista Paulista de Pediatria. 2019;**37**:161-165. DOI: 10.1590/1984-0462/;2019;37;2;00012

[26] Rybkin AV, Thoeni RF. Current concepts in imaging of appendicitis. Radiologic Clinics of North America.

2007;**45**(3):411-422. DOI: 10.1016/j.rcl.2007.04.003

[27] Nylund K, Ødegaard S, Hausken T, Folvik G, Lied GA, Viola I, et al. Sonography of the small intestine. World Journal of Gastroenterology: WJG. 2009;**15**(11):1319. DOI: 10.3748/wjg.15.1319

[28] Mostbeck G, Adam EJ, Nielsen MB, Claudon M, Clevert D, Nicolau C, et al. How to diagnose acute appendicitis: Ultrasound first. Insights Into Imaging. 2016;7(2):255-263. DOI: 10.1007/s13244-016-0469-6

[29] Jones MW, Lopez RA, Deppen JG. Appendicitis. Treasure Island, FL: StatPearls Publishing; 2021

[30] García-Marín A, Pérez-López M, Martínez-Guerrero E, Rodríguez-Cazalla L, Compañ-Rosique A. Microbiologic analysis of complicated and uncomplicated acute appendicitis. Surgical Infections. 2018;**19**(1):83-86. DOI: 10.1089/sur.2017.210

[31] Park NH, Oh HE, Park HJ, Park JY. Ultrasonography of normal and abnormal appendix in children. World Journal of Radiology. 2011;**3**:85-91. DOI: 10.4329/wjr.v3.i4.85

[32] Stackievicz R, Milner R, Werner M, Arnon S, Steiner Z. Follow-up ultrasonographic findings among children treated conservatively for uncomplicated acute appendicitis. Pediatric Radiology. 2022;**0**:1-12. DOI: 10.1007/s00247-022-05497-2

[33] Dirks K, Calabrese E, Dietrich CF, Gilja OH, Hausken T, Higginson A, et al. EFSUMB position paper: Recommendations for gastrointestinal ultrasound (GIUS) in acute appendicitis and diverticulitis. Ultraschall in der Medizin-European Journal of Ultrasound. 2019;**40**(02):163-175. DOI: 10.1055/a-0824-6952

[34] Harel S, Mallon M, Langston J, Blutstein R, Kassutto Z, Gaughan J. Factors contributing to nonvisualization of the appendix on ultrasound in children with suspected appendicitis. Pediatric Emergency Care. 2022;**38**(2):e678-e682. DOI: 10.1097/PEC.0000000000000239

[35] Kaneko K, Tsuda M. Ultrasound-based decision making in the treatment of acute appendicitis in children. Journal of Pediatric Surgery. 2004;**39**(9):1316-1320. DOI: 10.1016/j.jpedsurg.2004.05.011

[36] Lim HK, Lee WJ, Lee SJ, Namgung S, Lim JH. Focal appendicitis confined to the tip: Diagnosis at US. Radiology. 1996;**200**(3):799-801. DOI: 10.1148/radiology.200.3.8756934

[37] Moghadam MN, Salarzaei M, Shahraki Z. Diagnostic accuracy of ultrasound in diagnosing acute appendicitis in pregnancy: A systematic review and meta-analysis. Emergency Radiology. 2022;**29**:1, 437-12, 448. DOI: 10.1007/s10140-022-02021-9

[38] Lie G, Eleti S, Chan D, Roshen M, Cross S, Qureshi M. Imaging the acute abdomen in pregnancy: A radiological decision-making tool and the role of MRI. Clinical Radiology. 2022;**77**:639-649. DOI: 10.1016/j.crad.2022.05.021

[39] Mori T, Shin TS, Ong GY. High ascending retrocecal appendicitis in a pediatric patient detected by point-of-care ultrasound. Clinical Practice and Cases in Emergency Medicine. 2019;**3**(2):149. DOI: 10.5811/cpcem.2019.2.41682

[40] Prieto JM, Wang AW, Halbach J, Cauvi DM, Day JM, Gembicky M, et al.

Elemental, fatty acid, and protein composition of appendicoliths: Clues for understanding the pathogenesis of acute appendicitis. Scientific Reports. 2022;**12**:19764. DOI: 10.21203/rs.3.rs-1751015/v1

[41] Ranieri DM, Enzerra MD, Pickhardt PJ. Prevalence of appendicoliths detected at CT in adults with suspected appendicitis. American Journal of Roentgenology. 2021;**216**(3): 677-682. DOI: 10.2214/AJR.20.23149

[42] Babington EA. Complicated appendicitis in an adult patient. Ultrasound. 2022;**30**:1-5. DOI: 10.1177/1742271X221093

[43] Mosuka EM, Thilakarathne KN, Mansuri NM, Mann NK, Rizwan S, Mohamed AE, et al. A systematic review comparing nonoperative management to appendectomy for uncomplicated appendicitis in children. Cureus. 2021; **13**(10):e18901. DOI: 10.7759/cureus.18901

[44] Babington EA. Appendicoliths, the little giants: A narrative review. Radiography. 2023;**29**(1):1-7. DOI: 10.1016/j.radi.2022.09.006

[45] Bolmers MD, Bom WJ, Scheijmans JC, van Geloven AA, Boermeester M, Bemelman WA, et al. Accuracy of imaging in discriminating complicated from uncomplicated appendicitis in daily clinical practice. International Journal of Colorectal Disease. 2022;**37**:1-7. DOI: 10.1007/s00384-022-04173-z

[46] Levy S, Hiller N, Lev-Cohain N, Goldberg SN, Mizrahi I, Simanovsky N. Ultrasonographic features can predict outcome of conservative management of acute appendicitis in children. Emergency Radiology. 2022;**29**(1):59-65. DOI: 10.1007/s10140-021-01984-5

[47] Teixeira PALAG. Prospective observational study on acute appendicitis worldwide (POSAW). World Journal of Emergency Surgery : WJES. 2018;**13**:19. DOI: 10.1186/s13017-018-0179-0

[48] Goldin AB, Khanna P, Thapa M, McBroom JA, Garrison MM, Parisi MT. Revised ultrasound criteria for appendicitis in children improve diagnostic accuracy. Pediatric Radiology. 2011;**41**(8):993-999. DOI: 10.1007/s00247-011-2018-2

[49] Legault Kingstone L, Kielar AZ, McInnes M, Swan H. The potential value of adding colonic sonography to routine abdominal protocol in patients with active pain. Journal of Diagnostic Medical Sonography. 2011;**27**(3): 103-111. DOI: 10.1177/8756479311407198

[50] Blumfield E, Nayak G, Srinivasan R, Muranaka MT, Blitman NM, Blumfield A, et al. Journal club: Ultrasound for differentiation between perforated and nonperforated appendicitis in pediatric patients. American Journal of Roentgenology. 2013;**200**(5):957-962. DOI: 10.2214/AJR.12.9801

[51] Kidwai R, Sharma A. Acute perforated appendicitis: Clinical profile and analysis of risk factors. Journal of Nepalgunj Medical College. 2018;**16**(2): 13-15. DOI: 10.3126/jngmc.v16i2.24865

[52] Sanchez TR, Corwin MT, Davoodian A, Stein-Wexler R. Sonography of abdominal pain in children: Appendicitis and its common mimics. Journal of Ultrasound in Medicine. 2016;**35**(3):627-635. DOI: 10.7863/ultra.15.04047

[53] Majdawati A, Sari IGAPA. The evaluation of the sensitivity and specificity of ultrasound examination in

patients with suspected acute appendicitis. In: 4th International Conference on Sustainable Innovation 2020–Health Science and Nursing (ICoSIHSN 2020). The Netherlands: Atlantis Press; 2021. pp. 156-160. DOI: 10.2991/ahsr.k.210115.033

Section 2

Management of Complicated Appendicitis and Laparoscopic versus Open Surgery

Chapter 5

Perforated Appendicitis

Ibrahim Ethem Cakcak, Ahmet Orhan Sunar and Merve Yaren Kayabas

Abstract

Acute perforated appendicitis is a life-threatening disease because of sepsis. We will discuss the treatment options of acute perforated appendicitis. Is the surgical treatment necessary? How can we manage the patient without surgery in acute phase? Do we need also surgical treatment in the later time? What are the risks of surgery? What are the differences in surgical treatment options between the benign and malign causes of perforation? Do we need a multidisciplinary board to discuss the management options? Do we need laparoscopy always to decide even if the radiologic examination is negative? We can discuss the all conservative and surgical treatment options for acute perforated appendicitis.

Keywords: appendicitis, perforation, treatment

1. Introduction

Appendicitis is the most common cause of emergency surgery in the abdominal region caused by inflammation of the appendix, which is connected to the colon in the right lower quadrant [1, 2]. It occurs due to reasons such as infection or tumor [1]. It begins with a feeling of discomfort in the mid-abdominal region and progresses with pain localized to the right lower quadrant [1]. In addition to being more common in young ages and males, its overall incidence is 1 per 1000 persons per year [1, 3]. The presence of rupture complicates the appendix, while the absence of rupture can be defined as uncomplicated [1]. In this section, we aimed to provide up-to-date information on the approach in perforated appendicitis by reviewing the most recent studies in Pubmed and Google Scholar databases.

2. Causes

For many years, delay in the diagnosis or treatment of acute appendicitis was thought to be the cause of perforated appendicitis. In a multicenter study published in 2011, it was shown that delay in in-hospital treatment increases the risk of perforation in adults, and the cut-off time for over 65 s was 12 hours [4, 5]. In a meta-analysis conducted by Van Dijk in 2016, it was revealed that delaying the appendectomy until 24 hours after admission does not increase the risk of perforation [6]. Based on this study, the question of whether perforated appendicitis is caused by a delay in the treatment of appendicitis or arises as a different disease from appendicitis was again brought up for discussion. According to this second view, perforated appendicitis is a different entity from acute appendicitis, and patients already present with perforation findings at the time of admission, and early operation does not eliminate the risk of perforation. Although there are some recent studies showing that delay in the operation may be the cause of perforation, according to the existing literature, 24 hours after hospital admission is accepted as the safe time [7, 8]. Despite there is a study that states that the weakness of the longitudinal and circular muscles of the appendix makes perforation easier due to the anatomical structure of the appendix, this also explains why the tendency to perforation increases in the background of appendiceal neoplasia [9].

3. Diagnosis (blood neutrophil ratios, viewing etc.)

In a randomized controlled study on perforated appendicitis, the definition of perforation in the appendix was: (a) facilities in the abdomen, or (b) a hole in the appendix. In the same study, it was shown that the risk of intraperitoneal abscess development in the presence of purulent or gangrenous appendicitis is less than perforated appendicitis [10]. According to The American Association for the Surgery of Trauma (AAST) staging system, appendicitis is divided into five groups. Grade 1: acute inflamed, intact appendicitis, Grade 2: gangrenous intact appendicitis, Grade 3: perforated appendicitis with local contamination, Grade 4: perforated appendicitis with periappendiceal phlegmon or abscess, and Grade 5: perforated appendicitis with generalized peritonitis [11].

Since the presence of tachycardia is an indication of perforated appendicitis on admission to the hospital, it is recommended that these patients be given priority for early operation. The increase in the time between the onset of symptoms and admission to the hospital is also a risk factor for appendicitis perforation. It is thought that the time spent in the hospital after admission has no effect on appendicitis perforation [12]. In a study on the development of in-hospital perforation after admission to the hospital, it was shown that the risk of perforation increased 4.5 times in patients over the age of 46. The same study shows that leukocyte and neutrophil counts are also directly proportional to perforation [7]. A meta-analysis showed that the neutrophil/lymphocyte ratio alone is useful in both the diagnosis of acute appendicitis and the differentiation of complicated appendicitis. Accordingly, when the cut-off value in the neutrophil/lymphocyte ratio is above 8.8, complicated appendicitis can be predicted with 76.92% sensitivity and 100% specificity [13]. In the case of perforated appendicitis, regardless of the presence of an abscess, the number of WBCs has been shown to be higher than in non-perforated appendicitis [14]. Although there is a study showing that the male gender is associated with perforated appendicitis in the pediatric age group; In another study conducted in the adult age group, no relationship was found between gender and perforated appendicitis [15, 16].

In a multicenter prospective study comparing the use of Magnetic resonance imaging (MR) with the combined use of Computerized tomography (CT) and ultrasonography (USG) in the diagnosis of perforated appendicitis, it was observed that MR did not have any superiority in terms of sensitivity, specificity, positive predictive value and negative predictive value. The use of both MR and combined CT, ultrasonography evaluated about half of the perforated appendicitis as simple uncomplicated appendicitis. In this respect, it should be noted that the positive predictive value of imaging methods is generally low [17]. When ultrasonography is used alone, it is insufficient both in the diagnosis of appendicitis and in the differentiation of complicated and uncomplicated appendicitis. The sensitivity of CT in providing discrimination has been reported between 64 and 88% and specificity between 85 and 99% in different studies [18]. Among the CT findings, the findings with the highest specificity for complicated appendicitis are extraluminal appendicitis, abscess, presence of extraluminal air, contrast involvement defect in the appendix wall, and presence of ileus. Of these findings, only the presence of an involvement defect in the appendix wall has a moderate sensitivity with a rate of 59%. The sensitivity of others is below 50% [19]. It should be noted that CT without contrast has no place in both the diagnosis of acute appendicitis and the diagnosis of complicated appendicitis.

It has been observed that the incidence of appendicitis has increased during the Covid-19 pandemic process [20]. At the same time, it was observed that the symptoms of the patients worsened, and the perforation rate increased compared to the pre-pandemic period. As a result, the pandemic has caused delays in the diagnosis of appendicitis [4, 5].

4. Surgical vs. conservative approach

According to conservative approach, in the presence of appendicitis, treatment is done by intravenous antibiotics and surgery is postponed or not performed at all. While the conservative approach is almost avoided in the presence of generalized peritonitis due to perforated appendicitis, the clinical approach in perforated appendicitis with phlegmon or abscess is still controversial and there is no standard guideline recommendation. In a 2010 meta-analysis comparing the conservative approach to surgery, it was shown that the overall complication rate was lower in patients with the conservative approach. According to this meta-analysis, there were fewer wound infections, abdominal/pelvic abscesses, and ileus in the conservative treatment group [21]. In a recent meta-analysis involving randomized controlled trials, the hospital stay was 1 day shorter in the laparoscopic appendectomy group than in the conservatively followed group. In terms of general complications, it is seen that there is no difference between the two groups [22]. In the absence of equipment and an experienced team for laparoscopic surgery, conservative follow-up with perforated drainage should be preferred instead of open surgery for perforated appendicitis with phlegmon and abscess [23].

5. Open vs. laparoscopic surgery

Today, laparoscopic appendectomy is recommended over open appendectomy wherever there is equipment and an experienced team for both non-complicated and complicated appendicitis. McBurney is the most preferred incision in the open appendectomy method. However, in some patients or in rare cases, median or paramedian incisions may be preferred. In classical three-port laparoscopic appendectomy, left lower quadrant, suprapubic and umbilical trocars are used. A 5 mm umbilical trocar can be used if a 5 mm laparoscope is available. For closure of the appendix stump, linear stapler, simple intracorporeal ligation, extracorporeal prepared loop, or polymeric clip can be used, as well as ready-made industrial Endoloop. In the choice of surgical technique, classical three-port laparoscopic appendectomy should be preferred instead of single-port laparoscopic appendectomy because of both less postoperative pain and less wound infection [23]. In the presence of perforated appendicitis, the rate of conversion to open is significantly higher than those without perforation. In the presence of an abscess, the probability of opening increases 7.4 times, while it is 5.5 times in perforated appendicitis without an abscess [14].

6. Decision to wash or not

In patients who underwent appendectomy due to perforated appendicitis, it was observed that the operation time was prolonged when irrigation and aspiration were compared with only aspiration. However, peritoneal washing does not reduce the development of postoperative intra-abdominal abscess [24, 25]. Moreover, it is thought that peritoneal irrigation increases the risk of intra-abdominal abscess development in the pediatric age group [25].

Anderson et al. showed that irrigation with povidone-iodine after appendectomy moderately reduced the development of an intra-abdominal abscess. In this study, right upper, right lower quadrants and pelvis were washed after appendectomy using povidone-iodine diluted with SF at a ratio of 1:9, and after waiting for 1 minute, they were aspirated [26]. Povidone-iodine wash is promising for the development of intra-abdominal abscess after perforated appendicitis.

7. Whether to use a drain

According to the Cochrane meta-analysis, it is thought that the use of drains in patients undergoing surgery for complicated appendicitis has no effect on preventing intraperitoneal abscess [27]. There are also more recent studies that support this [28]. It has been shown that the use of drains has no effect in terms of wound infection [27]. There is also a study showing that the use of drains increases patient morbidity and health expenditures [29]. In addition, the use of drains causes prolongation of hospital stay [27].

According to a retrospective cohort study, if an intra-abdominal abscess develops due to perforated appendicitis, the length of hospital stay is prolonged and the overall cost increases by increasing hospitalization costs, medication costs and imaging costs [30]. For all these reasons, it is not recommended to place a drain during surgery for perforated appendicitis [23]. However, since there is no sufficient literature data on the use of drains in elderly patients, there are authors recommending drain placement as an expert recommendation [31].

8. Antibiotherapy use

Escherichia coli was the most grown bacteria in culture in both perforated and non-perforated acute appendicitis and was grown in all patients. The second most common bacterium is *Bacteroides fragilis*. However, Pseudomonas aeruginosa is the second most common bacteria growing in ASST Grade 5, that is, perforation with generalized peritonitis [32]. Considering this situation in the use of postoperative antibiotic therapy, regimens containing at least two drugs are generally preferred to cover these types. In a retrospective study conducted in the pediatric age group in postoperative antibiotherapy, the use of once-daily ceftriaxone and single-dose metronidazole, daily use of 4x1 ampicillin, 3x1 gentamicin and 4x1 clindamycin were compared, and it was shown that the use of single-dose ceftriaxone and metronidazole is a simple and sufficient combination and more cost-effective [33]. Although the use of piperacillin-tazobactam has come to the fore due to its antipseudomonal effect, retrospective cohort studies in the pediatric age group have shown that piperacillin-tazobactam combination is not superior to the ceftriaxone + metronidazole regimen. Therefore, routine use of antipseudomonal antibiotics is not recommended [34, 35]. It is recommended to start ceftriaxone and metronidazole after the diagnosis, before the operation and to continue after the operation [36]. However, it has been shown that the time from hospital admission to the initiation of antibiotic therapy does not increase the perforation rate [7].

9. Discharge

Postoperative discharge criteria of the patient include an afebrile course (<38°C for 24 hours, toleration by eating more than 50% of the normal diet for two consecutive meals, pain control with oral analgesics or ketorolac, benign examination, and mobilization). Prescribing oral antibiotics at discharge is still controversial. In a cohort study conducted in the pediatric population, oral antibiotics were not prescribed if there was no leukocytosis or left shift in the blood drawn on the day of discharge, and it was shown that the rate of surgical site infection or re-admission to the hospital did not increase in these patients [36].

10. What if it's a mucinous cyst?

When the pathologies of patients who underwent appendectomy with the diagnosis of acute appendicitis were examined retrospectively, the rate of appendiceal tumoral lesions was reported to be between 0.2% and 0.87%. Accumulation of mucinous acid in the abdominal cavity and associated complications may occur in low-grade appendiceal mucinous neoplasia, high-grade appendiceal mucinous neoplasia, or rupture of adenocarcinoma; this condition is defined as pseudomyxoma peritonei [37]. In the case of complicated appendicitis, when interval appendectomy was performed, the rate of appendiceal neoplasm was found to be higher in specimens than in early appendectomy. According to one review, the rate of neoplasia in interval appendectomy is 11%. Of these, 43% were appendiceal mucinous neoplasia, 29% were adenocarcinoma, 21% were neuroendocrine neoplasia, 13% were goblet cell carcinoma, and 20% were adenoma or serrated lesions [38]. The narrow lumen diameter of the appendix leads to premature occlusion of the lumen in the presence of neoplasm. In the presence of mucinous neoplasia, after lumen occlusion, the appendix becomes distended due to mucin and desquamated cells, which increases the tendency to appendicitis and perforation. In a retrospective study involving 3744 patients, the perforation rate was 80% in the presence of appendiceal neoplasm. Weakness of the longitudinal and circular muscle layer of the appendix causes the submucosa and peritoneum layers to be close to each other and the early spread of the lesion. Although perforation provides early clinical diagnosis and intervention, it causes intraperitoneal spread of tumor cells [9]. Some authors recommend a screening program with colonoscopy and CT to detect hidden pathologies, especially in patients over 40 years of age, if the decision to follow-up without surgery in complicated appendicitis is made. Despite this, appendiceal neoplasms rarely show signs before surgery, and therefore they are diagnosed either intraoperatively incidentally or by pathology in the postoperative period [38]. Previously, appendiceal mucinous neoplasms were treated with right hemicolectomy. Over time, it was seen that ileocolic lymph node dissection together with right hemicolectomy in appendiceal mucinous neoplasms with peritoneal metastases did not have a survival advantage and routine right hemicolectomy was abandoned. The concept of radical appendectomy has emerged in the treatment of these tumors, and it has been written that removal of the appendix with adjacent soft tissues and lymph nodes is sufficient. If necessary, it is recommended to switch from laparoscopic to open surgery [39]. In the presence of pseudomyxoma peritonei, the current treatment modality is cytoreductive surgery and hyperthermic intraperitoneal chemotherapy (HIPEC). In a recent cohort study, it was shown that HIPEC administered with mitomycin + cisplatin or oxaliplatin + fluorouracil/leucovorin combinations increased overall survival compared to the group that did no [40].

Author details

Ibrahim Ethem Cakcak[1*], Ahmet Orhan Sunar[2] and Merve Yaren Kayabas[3]

1 Faculty of Medicine, Department of General Surgery, Trakya University, Edirne, Turkey

2 Department of Gastroenterological Surgery, University of Health Sciences, Kartal Kosuyolu Higher Specialty Training and Research Hospital, Istanbul, Turkey

3 School of Medicine, Trakya University, Edirne, Turkey

*Address all correspondence to: ethemcakcak@hotmail.com

References

[1] Walter K. Acute Appendicitis. Journal of the American Medical Association. 2021;**326**(22):2339. DOI: 10.1001/jama.2021.20410

[2] Moris D, Paulson EK, Pappas TN. Diagnosis and Management of Acute Appendicitis in adults: A review. Journal of the American Medical Association. 2021;**326**(22):2299-2311. DOI: 10.1001/jama.2021.20502

[3] Téoule P, Laffolie J, Rolle U, Reissfelder C. Acute appendicitis in childhood and adulthood. Deutsches Ärzteblatt International. 2020;**117**(45):764-774. DOI: 10.3238/arztebl.2020.0764

[4] Cakcak İE, Türkyılmaz Z, Demirel T. Relationship between SIRI, SII values, and Alvarado score with complications of acute appendicitis during the COVID-19 pandemic. Ulus Travma Acil Cerrahi Derg. 2022;**28**(6):751-755. English. DOI: 10.14744/tjtes.2021.94580

[5] Busch M, Gutzwiller FS, Aellig S, Kuettel R, Metzger U, Zingg U. In-hospital delay increases the risk of perforation in adults with appendicitis. World Journal of Surgery. 2011;**35**(7):1626-1633. DOI: 10.1007/s00268-011-1101-z

[6] van Dijk ST, van Dijk AH, Dijkgraaf MG, Boermeester MA. Meta-analysis of in-hospital delay before surgery as a risk factor for complications in patients with acute appendicitis. The British Journal of Surgery. 2018;**105**(8):933-945. DOI: 10.1002/bjs.10873

[7] Hanson KA, Jacob D, Alhaj Saleh A, Dissanaike S. In-hospital perforation risk in acute appendicitis: Age matters. American Journal of Surgery. 2020;**219**(1):65-70. DOI: 10.1016/j.amjsurg.2019.05.015

[8] Cameron DB, Williams R, Geng Y, Gosain A, Arnold MA, Guner YS, et al. Time to appendectomy for acute appendicitis: A systematic review. Journal of Pediatric Surgery. 2018;**53**(3):396-405. DOI: 10.1016/j.jpedsurg.2017.11.042

[9] Lee WS, Choi ST, Lee JN, Kim KK, Park YH, Baek JH. A retrospective clinicopathological analysis of appendiceal tumors from 3,744 appendectomies: A single-institution study. International Journal of Colorectal Disease. 2011;**26**(5):617-621. DOI: 10.1007/s00384-010-1124-1

[10] St Peter SD, Sharp SW, Holcomb GW 3rd, Ostlie DJ. An evidence-based definition for perforated appendicitis derived from a prospective randomized trial. Journal of Pediatric Surgery. 2008;**43**(12):2242-2245. DOI: 10.1016/j.jpedsurg.2008.08.051

[11] Tominaga GT, Staudenmayer KL, Shafi S, Schuster KM, Savage SA, Ross S, et al. The American Association for the Surgery of Trauma grading scale for 16 emergency general surgery conditions: Disease-specific criteria characterizing anatomic severity grading. Journal of Trauma and Acute Care Surgery. 2016;**81**(3):593-602. DOI: 10.1097/TA.0000000000001127

[12] Kearney D, Cahill RA, O'Brien E, Kirwan WO, Redmond HP. Influence of delays on perforation risk in adults with acute appendicitis. Diseases of the Colon and Rectum. 2008;**51**(12):1823-1827. DOI: 10.1007/s10350-008-9373-6

[13] Hajibandeh S, Hajibandeh S, Hobbs N, Mansour M. Neutrophil-to-lymphocyte ratio predicts acute appendicitis and distinguishes between complicated and uncomplicated appendicitis: A systematic review and meta-analysis. American Journal of Surgery. 2020;**219**(1):154-163. DOI: 10.1016/j.amjsurg.2019.04.018

[14] Hester CA, Pickett M, Abdelfattah KR, Cripps MW, Dultz LA, Dumas RP, et al. Comparison of appendectomy for perforated appendicitis with and without abscess: A National Surgical Quality Improvement Program Analysis. The Journal of Surgical Research. 2020;**251**:159-167. DOI: 10.1016/j.jss.2019.12.054

[15] Zewdu D, Wondwosen M, Tantu T, Tilahun T, Teshome T, Hamu A. Predictors and management outcomes of perforated appendicitis in sub-Saharan African countries: A retrospective cohort study. Ann Med Surg (Lond). 2022;**80**:104194. DOI: 10.1016/j.amsu.2022.104194

[16] Zvizdic Z, Golos AD, Milisic E, Jonuzi A, Zvizdic D, Glamoclija U, et al. The predictors of perforated appendicitis in the pediatric emergency department: A retrospective observational cohort study. The American Journal of Emergency Medicine. 2021;**49**:249-252. DOI: 10.1016/j.ajem.2021.06.028

[17] Leeuwenburgh MM, Wiezer MJ, Wiarda BM, Bouma WH, Phoa SS, Stockmann HB, et al. Accuracy of MRI compared with ultrasound imaging and selective use of CT to discriminate simple from perforated appendicitis. The British Journal of Surgery. 2014;**101**(1):e147-e155. DOI: 10.1002/bjs.9350

[18] Bom WJ, Bolmers MD, Gans SL, van Rossem CC, van Geloven AAW, Bossuyt PMM, et al. Discriminating complicated from uncomplicated appendicitis by ultrasound imaging, computed tomography or magnetic resonance imaging: Systematic review and meta-analysis of diagnostic accuracy. BJS Open. 2021;**5**(2):zraa030. DOI: 10.1093/bjsopen/zraa030

[19] Kim HY, Park JH, Lee YJ, Lee SS, Jeon JJ, Lee KH. Systematic review and meta-analysis of CT features for differentiating complicated and uncomplicated appendicitis. Radiology. 2018;**287**(1):104-115. DOI: 10.1148/radiol.2017171260

[20] Orthopoulos G, Santone E, Izzo F, Tirabassi M, Pérez-Caraballo AM, Corriveau N, et al. Increasing incidence of complicated appendicitis during COVID-19 pandemic. American Journal of Surgery. 2021;**221**(5):1056-1060. DOI: 10.1016/j.amjsurg.2020.09.026

[21] Simillis C, Symeonides P, Shorthouse AJ, Tekkis PP. A meta-analysis comparing conservative treatment versus acute appendectomy for complicated appendicitis (abscess or phlegmon). Surgery. 2010;**147**(6):818-829. DOI: 10.1016/j.surg.2009.11.013

[22] Gavriilidis P, de Angelis N, Katsanos K, Di Saverio S. Acute Appendicectomy or conservative treatment for complicated appendicitis (Phlegmon or abscess)? A systematic review by updated traditional and cumulative meta-analysis. Journal of Clinical Medical Research. 2019;**11**(1):56-64. DOI: 10.14740/jocmr3672

[23] Di Saverio S, Podda M, De Simone B, Ceresoli M, Augustin G, Gori A, et al. Diagnosis and treatment of acute appendicitis: 2020 update of the WSES Jerusalem guidelines. World Journal of Emergency Surgery:

WJES. 2020;**15**(1):27. DOI: 10.1186/s13017-020-00306-3

[24] Bi LW, Yan BL, Yang QY, Cui HL. Peritoneal irrigation vs suction alone during pediatric appendectomy for perforated appendicitis: A meta-analysis. Medicine (Baltimore). 2019;**98**(50):e18047. DOI: 10.1097/MD.0000000000018047

[25] Siotos C, Stergios K, Prasath V, Seal SM, Duncan MD, Sakran JV, et al. Irrigation versus suction in laparoscopic appendectomy for complicated appendicitis: A meta-analysis. The Journal of Surgical Research. 2019;**235**:237-243. DOI: 10.1016/j.jss.2018.10.005

[26] Anderson KT, Putnam LR, Bartz-Kurycki MA, Hamilton EC, Yafi M, Pedroza C, et al. Povidone-iodine irrigation for pediatric perforated appendicitis may Be protective: A Bayesian pilot randomized controlled trial. Annals of Surgery. 2020;**271**(5):827-833. DOI: 10.1097/SLA.0000000000003398

[27] Li Z, Zhao L, Cheng Y, Cheng N, Deng Y. Abdominal drainage to prevent intra-peritoneal abscess after open appendectomy for complicated appendicitis. Cochrane Database Syst Rev. 2018;**5**(5):CD010168. DOI: 10.1002/14651858.CD010168.pub3. Update in: Cochrane Database Syst Rev. 2021 Aug 17;8:CD010168

[28] Ferguson DM, Anderson KT, Arshad SA, Garcia EI, Hebballi NB, Li LT, et al. Prophylactic intraabdominal drains do not confer benefit in pediatric perforated appendicitis: Results from a quality improvement initiative. Journal of Pediatric Surgery. 2021;**56**(4):727-732. DOI: 10.1016/j.jpedsurg.2020.06.031

[29] Chalya PL, Gilyoma JM, Mchembe M. Drain versus No drain after thyroidectomy: A prospective randomized clinical study. East and Central African Journal of Surgery. 2011;**16**(2):55-61

[30] Ferguson DM, Arshad SA, Avritscher EBC, Li LT, Austin MT, Kawaguchi AL, et al. Costs associated with postoperative intra-abdominal abscess in pediatric perforated appendicitis: A retrospective cohort study. Surgery. 2022;**172**(1):212-218. DOI: 10.1016/j.surg.2022.01.042

[31] Fugazzola P, Ceresoli M, Agnoletti V, Agresta F, Amato B, Carcoforo P, et al. The SIFIPAC/WSES/SICG/SIMEU guidelines for diagnosis and treatment of acute appendicitis in the elderly (2019 edition). World Journal of Emergency Surgery: WJES 2020;**15**(1):19. DOI: 10.1186/s13017-020-00298-0

[32] Abdul Jawad K, Qian S, Vasileiou G, Larentzakis A, Rattan R, Dodgion C, et al. Microbial epidemiology of acute and perforated appendicitis: A post-hoc analysis of an EAST multicenter study. The Journal of Surgical Research. 2022;**269**:69-75. DOI: 10.1016/j.jss.2021.07.026

[33] St Peter SD, Little DC, Calkins CM, Murphy JP, Andrews WS, Holcomb GW 3rd, et al. A simple and more cost-effective antibiotic regimen for perforated appendicitis. Journal of Pediatric Surgery. 2006;**41**(5):1020-1024. DOI: 10.1016/j.jpedsurg.2005.12.054

[34] Hamdy RF, Handy LK, Spyridakis E, Dona D, Bryan M, Collins JL, et al. Comparative effectiveness of ceftriaxone plus metronidazole versus anti-Pseudomonal antibiotics for perforated appendicitis in children. Surgical Infections. 2019;**20**(5):399-405. DOI: 10.1089/sur.2018.234

[35] Kashtan MA, Graham DA, Melvin P, Hills-Dunlap JL,

Anandalwar SP, Rangel SJ. Ceftriaxone with metronidazole versus piperacillin/Tazobactam in the management of complicated appendicitis in children: Results from a multicenter pediatric NSQIP analysis. Journal of Pediatric Surgery. 2022;**57**(10):365-372. DOI: 10.1016/j.jpedsurg.2021.11.009

[36] Theodorou CM, Lee SY, Lawrence Y, Saadai P, Hirose S, Brown EG. The utility of discharge antibiotics in pediatric perforated appendicitis without leukocytosis. The Journal of Surgical Research. 2022;**275**:48-55. DOI: 10.1016/j.jss.2022.01.024

[37] Koç C, Akbulut S, Akatlı AN, Türkmen Şamdancı E, Tuncer A, Yılmaz S. Nomenclature of appendiceal mucinous lesions according to the 2019 WHO classification of tumors of the digestive system. The Turkish Journal of Gastroenterology. 2020;**31**(9):649-657. DOI: 10.5152/tjg.2020.20537

[38] Peltrini R, Cantoni V, Green R, Lionetti R, D'Ambra M, Bartolini C, et al. Risk of appendiceal neoplasm after interval appendectomy for complicated appendicitis: A systematic review and meta-analysis. The Surgeon. 2021;**19**(6):e549-e558. DOI: 10.1016/j.surge.2021.01.010

[39] González-Moreno S, Sugarbaker PH. Radical appendectomy as an alternative to right colon resection in patients with epithelial appendiceal neoplasms. Surgical Oncology. 2017;**26**(1):86-90. DOI: 10.1016/j.suronc.2017.01.006

[40] Kusamura S, Barretta F, Yonemura Y, Sugarbaker PH, Moran BJ, Levine EA, et al. Peritoneal surface oncology group international (PSOGI) and the French National Registry of rare peritoneal surface malignancies (RENAPE). The role of Hyperthermic intraperitoneal chemotherapy in Pseudomyxoma Peritonei after Cytoreductive surgery. JAMA Surg. 2021;**156**(3):e206363. DOI: 10.1001/jamasurg.2020.6363

Chapter 6

Pediatric Complicated Appendicitis

Ndeye Aby Ndoye, Mamadou Mour Traoré, Aloïse Sagna, Aminah Oumou Rassoul Niane, Papa Alassane Mbaye, Florent Tshibwid A. Zeng, Oumar Ndour and Gabriel Ngom

Abstract

The objective of this study is to assess the frequency and the diagnostic features of complicated appendicitis in children and to search for factors that can predict the type of complication that may occur. We conducted a descriptive and analytical retrospective study over an 8-year period from July 1, 2010 to June 31, 2018, including children diagnosed and treated for the following complications. The data were collected at the pediatric surgery department of the Albert Royer Children's Hospital of Dakar. We collected 143 cases, representing 67.77% of all appendicular pathology. Encountered complications were 47.6% of abscesses, 42.6% of peritonitis, and 9.8% of appendicular mass. Appendicular syndrome was reported in 40.1% of cases, peritoneal irritation syndrome in 27.7% of cases, and occlusive syndrome in 6.2% of cases. Abdominal ultrasonography and plain X-ray allowed the diagnosis to be made in the majority of the cases. The analytical study showed that the clinical presentation and the white cell count can indicate the type of complication, unlike age and the duration of symptoms. In our practice, appendicular pathology often presents itself in complicated form. The clinical picture and the blood investigations' results can point to the type of complication.

Keywords: complicated appendicitis, children, appendicular abscess, appendicular mass, appendicular peritonitis, surgery

1. Introduction

Appendicular disease is one of the most common emergencies in visceral, pediatric surgery. It is a common disease, well known and falsely reputed to be benign. Appendicitis can lead to complications. The wide variation of symptoms contributes to delayed diagnosis and then to the occurrence of complications. The latter happens, such as appendicular abscess, appendicular mass, or peritonitis. These complicated appendicitis represent 30 to 70% of all appendicitis [1, 2]. They remain of great interest in our regions, where they are the most common presentation of appendicitis, with a high rate of morbidity [3–5]. Despite improvement of surgical techniques and implementation of medical management of pediatric complicated appendicitis, morbidity still reaches 5 to 14% [6]. We aimed to determine the frequency of complicated appendicitis, their diagnostic aspects, and the existence or not of predictors of complications type.

2. Patients and method

We conducted a retrospective study, descriptive and analytic, over eight years, from July 2010 to June 2018. We included patients aged from zero to 15 years diagnosed with appendicular mass, abscess, or peritonitis and managed in our pediatric surgery department, at Albert Royer National Children's Hospital Center, in Dakar. We collected 211 files of appendicular diseases. There were 89 boys and 60 girls. The mean age was 10.2 years, ranging from two to 15 years. In the descriptive part, we studied the frequency of complicated appendicitis, the complication type, and the positive diagnosis elements. In the analytic study, we tried to determine the existence of predictors of the kind of complication. Therefore, patients were subdivided into two groups according to age, with the first having patients aged five years and the second ranging from six to 15 years. We analyzed the following parameters with the type of complication: age, duration of symptoms, clinical presentation, and rate of white blood cells. The statistical method used was Fischer's exact test, with significance settled at p less than 0.05.

3. Results

3.1 Descriptive study

During the eight years of our study, we collected 143 cases of complicated appendicitis among the 211 cases of appendicitis, i.e., 67.77% of complicated forms. Among the 143 children with a complication, 68 had an abscess (47.6%), 61 a peritonitis (42.6%), and 14 had an appendicular mass (9.8%). A third of patients (37.5%) received at least one antibiotic before admission. We noted that 84.6% of them were referred from other medical institutions. Clinical presentations were grouped in appendicular syndrome (pain and tenderness in the right iliaca fossa, and cutaneous hyperesthesia), found in 57 patients, i.e., 40.1% of cases, peritoneal irritation syndrome (diffuse abdominal pain, generalized abdominal tenderness or contracture, and panful umbilical palpation) in 40 patients, i.e., 27.7% of cases, and ileus in nine patients, i.e., 6.2% of cases.

The mean white blood cell count for biology was 14,012 elements/$mm^{3,}$ and the mean CRP was 144 mg/l. Bacteriological examination identified a pathogen in 37 patients, and *Escherichia coli* was found in 62.1% of cases. Abdominal ultrasound allowed the diagnosis and determined the type of complication in 55.5% of cases. In 70% of children, a plain x-ray was realized; in 5.6% of patients, we needed an abdominal CT scan. A fourth of patients were managed using laparoscopy, as open surgery was used in the majority of case. The mean duration to surgery was 24 hours (6 – 30 hours).

Empiric antibiotics was made of three antibiotics, started from admission and continued until the postoperative period. Most used antibiotics were Matronidazole and Gentamicin each in 74.1% of cases, ampicillin in 66.1%, amoxicillin plus clavulanic acid in 8% of cases, third generation cephalosporins in 2.7% of cases and fluoroquinolones in 0.9%. A specific antibiotherapy was initiated in all patients for whom identified bacteria was resistant to molecules of empiric antibiotherapy. Hence, Ceftriaxone and Cefotaxime were respectively used in 3.6 and 2.7% of patients. Ciprofloxacin was used in 1.8% of cases, Ticarcillin and Imipenem were separately used each on a single patient, i.e. 0.9% of cases.

Postoperative complications occurred in 38% of patients, mainly represented by abdominal wall surgical site infection. Death occurred in 2.4% of cases.

3.2 Analytic study

3.2.1 Age/type of complication

Table 1 shows the repartition of type of complication according to patients' age. Statistical analysis of these variables did not find a significant difference between age and type of complication ($p = 0,348$).

3.3 Symptoms duration/type of complication

Symptoms duration was given in 122 patients with a mean of 4 days. It was less than 2 days in 13 patients (10.7%). In 49 patients (40.2%), it was between 2 and 5 days; in 60 patients (49.2%), it was more than 5 days. Statistical analysis between symptoms duration and type of complication did not find any significant difference ($p = 0.71$).

3.4 Clinical presentation/type of complication

Clinical presentation and type of complication analysis showed that appendicular syndrome was found in patients with appendicular abscesses. However, peritoneal irritation syndrome and ileus were essentially noted in patients with peritonitis from perforated appendicitis. Then, there was a significant link between clinical presentation and type of complication, $p = 0.003$.

3.5 White blood cells count/type of complication

In 9 patients, i.e. 6.3%, the WBC were less than 10,000 elements/mm^3, in 12 patients, i.e. 8.5%, it was between 10,000 and 12,000, in 24 patients, i.e. 17%, it was between 12,000 and 15,000, and in 94 patients, i.e. 66%, it was at least 15,000 elements/mm. In cases of peritonitis or appendicular abscess, 75, and 72%, respectively, as shown in **Table 2**. Analysis of white blood cell count and type of complication showed a significant link ($p = 0.002$).

Age ranges (in years)	Diagnosis			Total
	Appendicular Abscess (%)	Appendicular peritonitis (%)	Appendicular mass (%)	
[0 – 5]	2 (40.0)	3 (60)	0 (0.0)	5 (100)
[6–10]	25 (45.5)	23 (41.8)	7 (12.7)	55 (100)
[11–15]	26 (50.0)	22 (42.3)	4 (7.7)	52 (100)
Total	53 (47.3)	48 (42.9)	11 (9.8)	112 (100)

Table 1.
Type of complication according to age.

Symptoms duration (in days)	Diagnosis			Total
	Appendicular Abscess (%)	Appendicular peritonitis (%)	Appendicular mass (%)	
< 2	6 (60,0)	3 (30)	1 (10.0)	10 (100)
2 - 5	18 (47.4)	20 (52.6)	0 (0.0)	38 (100)
> 5	17 (36.2)	22 (46.8)	8 (17.0)	47 (100)
Total	41 (43.2)	45 (47.4)	9 (9.5)	112 (100)

Table 2.
Type of complication according to symptoms duration.

4. Discussion

Complicated appendicitis represents 30 to 60% of all pediatric appendicitis, as stated by many authors [7–9]. For some, it represents an entirely different entity, not necessarily from uncomplicated appendicitis [7, 10, 11]. Its frequency in our series was 67.77%, frankly more than data reported in the literature. This high frequency of complicated appendicitis with delayed presentation could be explained by delayed diagnosis due to auto-medication, lack of qualified health workers in peripheral medical institutions, and the abusive use of antibiotics. A third of our patients already received antibiotics prior to diagnosis of appendicitis.

The symptoms duration was between 2 and 5 in half of the cases. After analysis, this does not impact the type of complication ($p = 0.71$). In the case of complicated appendicitis, peritoneal irritation syndrome and ileus favored the presence of peritonitis, while appendicular syndrome was oriented towards appendicular abscess or mass ($p = 0.003$). These orientation elements could allow the creation of diagnostic guidelines. Such guidelines, like acute appendicitis, aim to ease the diagnosis and implement better therapeutic strategies for each case [12]. If a detailed clinical examination can diagnose uncomplicated appendicitis, the diagnosis of type of complication is more difficult in the case of a complicated one. However, it is crucial for adapted management. Biological data are more objective and reproducible [13, 14], but their value should be correlated to the clinical presentation [15]. So, some factors, such as fibrinogen, predict perforated appendicitis [16]. Most of our patients had a white blood cell count of at least 15,000 elements/mm. The statistical analysis showed a significant link between white blood cell count and the type of complication. In our series, a link between CRP and type of complication was not investigated to avoid bias since only 42% of patients had this dosage realized before administering antibiotics. Management of appendicular disease benefited from improvement of minimally invasive surgery. However, in our context, open surgery is still mainly practiced. The use of laparoscopy for management of these diseases is difficult due to underequipement and organizational reasons for emergency management. Its use would allow decrease of surgical site infection. High mortality in our series, for other African studies may be linked to delayed diagnosis, automedication, and low socioeconomic level.

5. Limitations

Limitations of our studies are due to its retrospective nature: inflammatory investigations were not done in all patient before antibiotics were started. Patients referred to other hospitals for not working operating room were not included in our study. A third of patients received antibiotics prior to admission, as the remaining received their first dose on admission day.

6. Conclusion

Complicated appendicitis is a spectrum of appendicular pathology which is still not well understood despite numerous studies. It is a specific entity, not always resulting from natural history of acute appendicitis. In our practice, appendicitis is frequently managed when complicated such as an abscess or peritonitis. The clinical presentation and white blood cell count gave orientation for the type of complication, while the patient's age and symptoms' duration did not. In our context, morbidity and mortality of this disease remains a challenge.

Author details

Ndeye Aby Ndoye[1*], Mamadou Mour Traoré[2], Aloïse Sagna[1], Aminah Oumou Rassoul Niane[1], Papa Alassane Mbaye[1], Florent Tshibwid A. Zeng[1], Oumar Ndour[3] and Gabriel Ngom[1]

1 Department of Pediatric Surgery, Albert Royer National Children's Hospital Centre, Cheikh Anta Diop University, Dakar, Senegal

2 Department of Anesthesia and Intensive Care, Albert Royer National Children's Hospital Centre, Cheikh Anta Diop University, Dakar, Senegal

3 Department of Pediatric Surgery, Aristide Le Dantec University Teaching Hospital, Cheikh Anta Diop University, Dakar, Senegal

*Address all correspondence to: aby_ndoye@yahoo.fr

References

[1] Hafid M, Erraji M, Kisra M, Ettayebi F. Appendicites aigues de l'enfant de moins de 5ans: étude diagnostique. Journal of Pédiatrics and Childcare. 2009;**22**:14-18

[2] Sapin E, Joyeux L. Appendicite aigue de l'enfant en 2008. Archives de Pédiatrie. 2008;**15**:559-561

[3] Ndour O, Faye Fall A, Mbaye PA, Ndoye NA, Seck NF, Ngom G, et al. Complications de l'appendicectomie chez l'enfant (Revue Africaine de Chirurgie et Spécialités). African Journal of Surgery and Specialities. 2015;**1**:18-23

[4] Farthouat P, Fall O, Goug Bemy MO, Sow A, Millo A, Dieng D, et al. Appendicectomie en milieu tropical: Etude prospective à l'Hôpital Principal de Dakar. Tropical Medicine. 2005;**65**:549-553

[5] Rantomalala HYN, Rakotondrabe JB. RA-Jaonarivony T. Les complications postopératoires d'une appendicectomie classique. Méd Afr Noire. 2005;**52**(1):56-60

[6] Podevin G, Barussaud M, Leclair M-D, Heloury Y. Appendicite et péritonite appendiculaire de l'enfant. EMC Pédiatrie. 2005;**2**:211-219

[7] Anderson Jamie E, Stephen Bickler W, David C, Chang DC, Mark A, Talamini MA. Examining a common disease with unknown etiology: Trends in epidemiology and surgical Management of Appendicitis in California, 1995-2009. World Journal of Surgery. 2012;**36**(12):2787-2794

[8] Bratton SL, Haberkern CM, Waldhausen JH. Acute appendicitis risks of complications: Age and Medicaid insurance. Pediatrics. 2000;**106**:75-78

[9] Xuan-Binh P, Veronica FC, Dennis YK, Blake R, Amyh K, De Virgilio C, et al. Factors predictive of complicated appendicitis in children. The Journal of Surgical Research. 2016;**206**:62-66

[10] David RF, Morris A, Koepsell T, Dellinger P. Has misdiagnosis of appendicitis decreased over time? A population-based analysis JAMA. 2001;**286**(14):1748-1753

[11] Marudanayagam R, Williams GT, Rees BI. Review of the pathological results of 2660 appendicectomy specimens. Journal of Gastroenterology. 2006;**41**(8):745-749

[12] Podevin G, de Vries P, Lardy H, Garignon C, Petit T, Azzis O. Intérêt d'un protocole simple pour améliorer l'utilisation des examens complémentaires dans le diagnostic d'appendicite chez l'enfant. Journal of Visceral Surgery. 2017;**154**(4):253-260

[13] Zouari M, Abid I, Sallami S, Guitouni A, Ben Dhaou M, Jallouli M. Predictive factors of complicated appendicitis in children. American Journal of Emergency Medicine. 2016;**25**:109-113

[14] Ramon RG, Van Den Boom LA. A scoring system to predict the severity of appendicitis in children. The Journal of Surgical Research. 2016;**200**:452-459

[15] Rodiere M, Zebiche H. Indicateurs des marqueurs biologiques d'infection en situation d'urgence. Archies in Pédiatrics. 2002;**9**(2):219-222

[16] Alvarez-Alvarez FA, Maciel-Gutierrez VM, Rocha-Muñoz AD, Lujan JH, Ploneda-Valancia CF. Diagnostic value of serum fibrinogen as a predictive factor for complicated appendicitis (perforated). A cross-sectional study. International Journal of Surgery. 2016;**25**:109-113

Chapter 7

Treatment of Complicated Appendicitis

Pratima Gautam, Prakash Mainali, Sandeep Bhattarai and Sunil Kumar Das

Abstract

Acute complicated appendicitis is defined as the presence of any of the four findings; visible hole, diffuse fibrinopurulent exudate, intra-abdominal abscess, and extraluminal fecalith. Different scoring systems such as appendicitis severity index (APSI) use different clinical and radiological parameters to diagnose complicated appendicitis. Surgical treatment is preferred over conservative treatment. Though previous studies showed open method is best for complicated appendicitis, present studies have shown that laparoscopic method also has similar results as open in terms of development of surgical site infection (superficial, deep or organ space), post-operative prolonged ileus or postoperative hospital stay. Intraoperatively irrigation of the peritoneal cavity is preferred over suction only method but is not statistically significant. Drain placement is not recommended. Postoperative antibiotics should be given for 3–6 days. Tazobactam—Piperacillin is an antibiotic of choice. Postoperative complications include surgical site infection, intra-abdominal abscess, and adhesive intestinal obstruction.

Keywords: appendicitis, complicated, irrigation, suction, intra-abdominal abscess

1. Introduction

Complicated appendicitis (CA) is a controversial topic in acute appendicitis. The definition is not standard and universal, diagnosis is difficult, management is not definite with high chance of complication, and worse outcome with increased cost. This chapter aims to summarize and standardize the topic.

2. Definition

Cameron et al. defined CA in the pediatric population as presence of any of the four findings: visible hole, diffuse fibrinopurulent exudate, intra-abdominal abscess, and extraluminal fecalith [1]. Many have accepted perforated appendicitis, gangrenous appendicitis, and suppurative appendicitis as CA [2, 3].

Grade	Laparoscopic findings
0	Normal looking appendix
1	Hyperemia and edema
2	Fibrinous exudate
3A	Segmental necrosis
3B	Base necrosis
4A	Abscess
4B	Regional peritonitis
5	Diffuse peritonitis

Table 1.
Grading of complicated appendicitis [4].

Type of inflammation	Histological criteria
Appendicitis with minor inflammation	Focal acute inflammation in the mucosa
Phlegmonous	Polymorphonuclear infiltration of the entire appendiceal wall without evidence of necrosis
Gangrenous	Phlegmonous type but presence of necrosis
Appendicitis with perforation	Rupture of the appendiceal wall to the serosal surface
Periappendicitis	Inflammation in the serosa, eventually affecting the longitudinal muscular layer

Table 2.
Histological criteria of appendicitis [6].

Maxime et al. did a video survey analysis in 2019 in a classification of appendicitis on the basis of laparoscopic findings given by Gomez et al. in 2012 with 85% concordance between surgeons hence good reproducibility which is shown in **Table 1** [4, 5].

Histological grading was given by Pieper in 1981 which is shown in the **Table 2** [6]. Later in 2022 Kadi et al. showed different histological findings in acute appendicitis recorded as acute hemorrhagic appendicitis, acute appendicitis with gangrene, acute necrotizing appendicitis, acute appendicitis with perforation, and acute suppurative appendicitis. The most common was acute suppurative appendicitis and least common was acute hemorrhagic appendicitis [7].

The incidence of perforated appendicitis ranges from 8.7 to 12.6% [7, 8] and gangrenous appendicitis is 2.55% [7]. There is a tendency of increasing incidence of CA in extremes of age [9]. During COVID the management of appendicitis was changed as non-operative management was mostly adopted which had some impact on the increase in incidence of complicated appendicitis due to delay in treatment. Many studies have shown increased incidence of complicated appendicitis in adults as well as children during COVID [2, 10].

It may be thought that CA can arise when uncomplicated appendicitis is not managed. However a study done by Livingstone showed that there is no relation between negative appendectomy and perforation rate suggesting that perforated and non-perforated appendicitis have different pathophysiology [11]. Clinical presentation of CA can vary from right lower quadrant pain to generalized abdominal pain and examination findings can vary from right lower quadrant tenderness to features of generalized tenderness [12].

3. Diagnosis

Diagnosing CA can be challenging at times. Alvarado scoring system is used initially and then ultrasound of abdomen and pelvis is done. Ultrasound is a good radiological tool to differentiate complicated from uncomplicated appendicitis. Increased appendiceal diameter, periappendiceal fat inflammation, presence of an appendicolith and a suspected perforation are discriminatory markers [13]. WSES guidelines say to perform computed tomography when the ultrasound findings are inconclusive or in a patient >40 years of age [14]. The overall CT sensitivity, specificity, and accuracy for differentiation of complicated from uncomplicated appendicitis were 87.2%, 75.7%, and 81.1%, respectively. The most sensitive CT findings of complicated appendicitis were mucosal enhancement defect and moderate-to-severe periappendiceal fat stranding [13]. Phlegmon, fluid collection, extraluminal appendicolith, periappendiceal air, and small bowel dilatation had specificity of 98.1–100% [3].

The CA must be distinguished from uncomplicated appendicitis and at times it is challenging. Scoring system is created to distinguish CA from uncomplicated appendicitis to help manage the cases. Atema et al. created a scoring system using clinical and imaging features. Clinical and radiological features included age, body temperature, duration of symptoms, white blood cell counts, C-reactive protein level, and presence of extraluminal free air, periappendiceal fluid, and appendicolith shown in **Table 3** [15].

Features/points scored	Clinical and CT features	Clinical and ultrasound features
Age >/= 45 yrs	2	2
Body temperature		
</= 37	0	0
37.1–37.9	2	2
>/= 38.0	4	4
Duration of symptoms >/= 48 h	2	2
WBC count >13,000/dl	2	2
C-reactive protein (mg/l)		
<50	0	0
51–100	2	4
>100	3	5
Extraluminal free air on imaging	5	—
Periappendiceal fluid on imaging	2	2
Appendicolith on imaging	2	2
Maximum score	22	19

Table 3.
Clinical and radiological scoring for complicated appendicitis [15].

SAGS score	Intraoperative findings
0	No appendicitis
1	Simple appendicitis (any of the following)
	I. Infected appendix
	II. Thickened appendix
	III. Serous free fluid
2	Purulent appendicitis (any of the following)
	I. Pus localized to right iliac fossa
	II. Right paracolic gutter
	III. Pelvis
3	Purulent appendicitis with four quadrant contamination
4	Perforated appendix (any of the following)
	I. Free fecalith, feces
	II. Fecal staining
	III. Visible hole in appendix

Table 4.
SAGS score [23].

Hyponatremia is regarded as a risk factor for development of CA [16]. According to Oba et al. old age, larger body mass index, smoking, and medication with antidiabetic drugs, oral corticosteroids, oral antiplatelet drugs, and oral anticoagulant drugs are independent risk factors for CA [17]. Duration of chief complaint, history of constipation, having history of visit to health facilities without surgical intervention for their current problem and fever are also considered as risk factors for CA [18]. Pelvic appendix may be a new risk factor associated with CA [19]. However appendix length was not considered as a risk factor [20].

Different scoring systems predict the severity of appendicitis. One of the commonly used scoring systems, the Alvarado scoring system helps to diagnose acute appendicitis but is not helpful to grade the severity of acute appendicitis [21]. Appendicitis severity index (APSI) uses different clinical and radiological parameters to diagnose complicated appendicitis. Three clinical (age $\geq$ 52 years, body temperature $\geq$ 37.5°C, duration of symptoms $\geq$48 h) and four computed tomography (CT) findings (appendix diameter $\geq$ 14 mm, presence of periappendiceal fluid, extraluminal air, perityphlitic abscess) are used and score of $\geq$4 is predicted as complicated appendicitis [22]. Another scoring system called Sunshine appendicitis grading system score (SAGS) uses intraoperative findings to grade the severity of appendicitis shown in **Table 4** [23].

4. Management

The optimum management of CA is a subject of controversy. Conservative treatment is one of the treatment options for acute appendicitis. In conservative treatment patients are given antibiotics and kept nil per oral and observed till the pain subsides. It was majorly performed before the surgery was practiced and during the COVID. The effective rate of conservative treatment in uncomplicated appendicitis is 95.2% and in complicated appendicitis is 83.4%. The complication rate of conservative treatment in uncomplicated appendicitis is 3.5% and in complicated appendicitis is 12.1% [24].

A meta-analysis conducted by Simillis et al. discussed conservative management of complicated appendicitis has been associated with decreased complication and reoperation compared to acute appendectomy and has almost similar hospital stay [25]. Delayed operative management may be associated with a reduction in the need of extended resection appendectomy, shorter operative time, and a trend toward reduced mortality. But it may also be associated with an increased length of in-hospital stay and short-term morbidity [26]. Similarly in pediatric age group appendicular abscess and perforated appendix are better managed with non-operative management, conversely free perforated appendix showed lower complication rate and readmission when treated with surgery [27]. However, a study conducted by Vasos et al. in 2019 states immediate surgery is associated with shorter duration of hospital stay, whereas postoperative complication was not affected by treatment of choice [28]. Most of the patients with appendicoliths had to undergo surgery despite being on antibiotics [29] and CA had more chances of having appendicolith than uncomplicated appendicitis [30]. Endoscopic therapy of acute appendicitis helps to clear appendicolith by stenting appendix and is being considered as a treatment option in case of uncomplicated appendicitis but study for its role in complicated appendicitis is yet to be performed [31, 32].

Surgery was regarded as gold standard treatment for more than a century because of its low incidence of postoperative complications, early recovery, and short hospital stay. Emergency surgery is mandated when the patient develops generalized peritonitis. Surgery is also considered a better option in pregnancy and it is associated with a lower rate of maternal and fetal complications. Failed non-operative management was associated with higher maternal and fetal complication rate [33]. Surgery is the only option with no scope for conservative treatment for complicated appendicitis caused by foreign body ingestion such as toothpick [34].

Open surgery had been the gold standard until the last 20 years when laparoscopic appendectomy became a preferred option for most of the surgeons because of its advantages like less pain, lower wound infection rate, and short recovery period [35]. However laparoscopic appendectomy has similar intra-abdominal abscess rate, readmission, and reoperation rate [36]. According to Jung Oh et al. single incision laparoscopic appendectomy (SILA) is also a feasible option for complicated appendicitis as there was no difference in operative time and postoperative infectious complication but hospital stay and drain insertion rate was significantly lower compared to conventional laparoscopic appendectomy [37]. Though laparoscopic appendectomy is gold standard, in low and middle human development index countries like Nepal open appendectomy is still more commonly practiced. Also some studies have shown that open appendectomy is preferred for CA. Foster et al. showed that open surgery is preferred in patients with intra-abdominal abscess [38].

Sun et al. showed that peritoneal irrigation is associated with lower rate of intra-abdominal abscess, shorter hospital stay, and earlier anal exsufflation compared to suction only group in patients with CA [39]. But these findings were not significant according to a meta-analysis. There is increased intraoperative time with irrigation. Also there is an increased chance of intra-abdominal abscess with irrigation in the pediatric population [40]. Hence peritoneal irrigation though preferred has no added advantage in preventing development of intra-abdominal abscess and surgical site infection in both adult and pediatric population [14]. Drain placement is not shown to decrease the rate of intra-abdominal abscess formation. Hence drain is not necessary after appendectomy; rather it can increase risk of postoperative complications such as fistula, surgical site infection (SSI), bowel obstruction, ileus, and length of hospital stay [41, 42].

Post-operative antibiotics are indicated in case of CA. However, the duration is not specified. Less than or equal to 5 days of antibiotics is seen to have more intra-abdominal abscess hence >5 days of antibiotics is preferred. But the duration of antibiotics can be individualized based on the response of the patient [43]. Panshin et al. recommended 3–6 days of antibiotics [44]. Longer duration of antibiotics was not associated with a low rate of complication [45]. For the pediatric population antibiotics can be stopped before postoperative day 7, on the day of discharge [46].

Antibiotics should be chosen wisely for CA as there is significant increased risk of complication in co-amoxiclav resistant E.coli. Also complication rate is increased when pseudomonas is not covered [47]. Routine intraoperative bacterial culture can be done to select antibiotics of choice [48]. Piperacillin—Tazobactam is considered antibiotic of choice to cover the resistant group [49]. Triple regimen consisting of ampicillin, metronidazole, and gentamicin and monotherapy consisting of amoxycillin and clavulanic acid can be the alternative antibiotics [50].

There is a high chance of postoperative complication associated with complicated appendicitis. Postoperative complications include surgical site infection (SSI), intra-abdominal abscess, adhesive intestinal obstruction. SSI can occur in as high as 30.4% and serious complications like intra-abdominal collection and adhesive intestinal obstruction can occur in 13.48% cases [51]. Compared to uncomplicated appendicitis, complicated appendicitis have longer operative duration, greater blood loss, longer hospital stay [52].

5. Conclusions

Complicated appendicitis should be treated with surgery. Intraoperatively irrigation of the peritoneum should be done. Drain is not recommended and postoperatively antibiotics should be continued till 3–6 days.

Conflict of interest

No.

Notes

Pratima Gautam = https://orcid.org/0000-0003-3939-3705
Prakash Mainali = https://orcid.org/0000-0001-6307-5497
Sunil Kumar Das = https://orcid.org/000-0002-6568-5149
Sandeep Bhattarai https://orcid.org/0000-0002-7907-6766

Author details

Pratima Gautam[1*], Prakash Mainali[2], Sandeep Bhattarai[3] and Sunil Kumar Das[3]

1 Gorkha Hospital, Gorkha, Nepal

2 Tribhuvan University Teaching Hospital, Kathmandu, Nepal

3 Patan Academy of Health Sciences, Kathmandu, Nepal

*Address all correspondence to: gautampratima333@gmail.com

References

[1] Cameron DB, Anandalwar SP, Graham DA, Melvin P, Serres SK, Dunlap JL, et al. Development and implications of an evidence-based and public health-relevant definition of complicated appendicitis in children. Annals of Surgery 2020;**271**:962-968. 10.1097/SLA.0000000000003059

[2] Pogorelić Z, Anand S, Žuvela T, Singh A, Križanac Z, Krishnan N. Incidence of complicated appendicitis during the COVID-19 pandemic versus the pre-pandemic period: A systematic review and Meta-analysis of 2782 Pediatric appendectomies. Diagnostics (Basel) 2022;202212. 10.3390/diagnostics12010127

[3] Iamwat J, Teerasamit W, Apisarnthanarak P, Noppakunsomboon N, Kaewlai R. Predictive ability of CT findings in the differentiation of complicated and uncomplicated appendicitis: A retrospective investigation of 201 patients undergone appendectomy at initial admission. Insights Into Imaging 2021;**12**:143. 10.1186/s13244-021-01086-3

[4] Gomes CA, Nunes TA, Fonseca Chebli JM, Junior CS, Gomes CC. Laparoscopy grading system of acute appendicitis: New insight for future trials. Surgical Laparoscopy, Endoscopy & Percutaneous Techniques 2012;**22**:463-466. 10.1097/SLE.0b013e318262edf1

[5] Mariage M, Sabbagh C, Grelpois G, Prevot F, Darmon I, Regimbeau J-M. Surgeon's definition of complicated appendicitis: A prospective video survey study. Euroasian Journal of Hepatogastroenterology 2019;**9**:1-4. 10.5005/jp-journals-10018-1286

[6] Pieper R. Acute appendicitis: A study of its pathogenesis, clinical features and histopathology. In: Postgraduate Medical Thesis. Stockholm: Karolinska Institute; 1981. pp. v-5

[7] Kadi M, Nasr A, Shabkah AA, Alnahari R, Alhawi A, Alyamani R, et al. Histopathological examination of cases with acute appendicitis, A retrospective study at King Abdulaziz University Hospital, Jeddah, Saudi Arabia, Annals of Medical Surgery (Lond) 2022;**81**:104401. 10.1016/j.amsu.2022.104401

[8] Gofrit ON, Abu-Dalu K. Perforated appendicitis in the child: Contemporary experience. The Israel Medical Association Journal. 2001;**3**:262-265

[9] Körner H, Söndenaa K, Söreide JA, Andersen E, Nysted A, Lende TH, et al. Incidence of acute nonperforated and perforated appendicitis: Age-specific and sex-specific analysis. World Journal of Surgery 1997;**21**:313-317. 10.1007/s002689900235

[10] Kariya A, Krutsri C, Singhatas P, Sumritpradit P, Thampongsa T, Lertsitthichai P, et al. Incidence of complicated appendicitis during the COVID-19 pandemic: A systematic review and meta-analysis. International Journal of Surgical Open 2022;**45**:100512. 10.1016/j.ijso.2022.100512

[11] Livingston EH, Woodward WA, Sarosi GA, Haley RW. Disconnect between incidence of nonperforated and perforated appendicitis: Implications for pathophysiology and management. Annals of Surgery 2007;**245**:886-892. 10.1097/01.sla.0000256391.05233.aa

[12] Dagne H, Abebaw T-A. Characteristics of patients presented with complicated appendicitis in Adama, Ethiopia: A cross-sectional study. Open Access Emerg Medicine 2022;**14**:573-580. 10.2147/OAEM.S383550

[13] Rawolle T, Reismann M, Minderjahn MI, Bassir C, Hauptmann K, Rothe K, et al. Sonographic differentiation of complicated from uncomplicated appendicitis. The British Journal of Radiology 2019;**92**:20190102. 10.1259/bjr.20190102

[14] Di Saverio S, Podda M, De Simone B, Ceresoli M, Augustin G, Gori A, et al. Diagnosis and treatment of acute appendicitis: 2020 update of the WSES Jerusalem guidelines. World Journal of Emergency Surgery : WJES 2020;**15**:27. 10.1186/s13017-020-00306-3

[15] Atema JJ, van Rossem CC, Leeuwenburgh MM, Stoker J, Boermeester MA. Scoring system to distinguish uncomplicated from complicated acute appendicitis. The British Journal of Surgery 2015;**102**:979-990. 10.1002/bjs.9835

[16] Symeonidis NG, Pavlidis ET, Psarras KK, Stavrati K, Nikolaidou C, Marneri A, et al. Preoperative hyponatremia indicates complicated acute appendicitis. Surgery Research Practise 2022;**2022**:1836754. 10.1155/2022/1836754

[17] Oba T, Yamada T, Matsuda A, Otani M, Matsuda S, Ohta R, et al. Patient backgrounds and short-term outcomes of complicated appendicitis differ from those of uncomplicated appendicitis. Annals of Gastroenterological Surgery 2022;6:273-281. 10.1002/ags3.12523

[18] Bayissa BB, Miressa F, Abulkadir A, Fekadu G. Predictors of complicated appendicitis among patients presented to public referral hospitals in Harari region, Eastern Ethiopia: A case-control study. Surgery in Practice and Science 2022;**9**:100072. 10.1016/j.sipas.2022.100072

[19] Koh H, Yang H, Cho K, Jung YY, Chang YS, Kim DH, et al. Risk factor leading to complicated appendicitis: Pelvic position of the appendix. Journal of The Korean Society of Emergency Medicine. 2021;**32**:134-142

[20] Dibekoğlu C. Does the length matter in acute appendicitis for the perforation risk?: A retrospective cohort study. Medicine 2022;**101**:e32001. 10.1097/MD.0000000000032001

[21] Chung PHY, Dai K, Yang Z, Wong KKY. Validity of Alvarado score in predicting disease severity and postoperative complication in pediatric acute appendicitis. World Journal of Pediatric Surgery 2019;**2**:e000003. 10.1136/wjps-2018-000003

[22] Avanesov M, Wiese NJ, Karul M, Guerreiro H, Keller S, Busch P, et al. Diagnostic prediction of complicated appendicitis by combined clinical and radiological appendicitis severity index (APSI). European Radiology 2018;**28**:3601-3610. 10.1007/s00330-018-5339-9

[23] Reid F, Choi J, Williams M, Chan S. Prospective evaluation of the sunshine appendicitis grading system score. ANZ Journal of Surgery 2017;**87**:368-371. 10.1111/ans.13271

[24] Yang Z, Sun F, Ai S, Wang J, Guan W, Liu S. Meta-analysis of studies comparing conservative treatment with antibiotics and appendectomy for acute appendicitis in the adult. BMC Surgery 2019;**19**:110. 10.1186/s12893-019-0578-5

[25] Simillis C, Symeonides P, Shorthouse AJ, Tekkis PP. A meta-analysis comparing conservative treatment versus acute appendectomy for complicated appendicitis (abscess or phlegmon). Surgery 2010;**147**:818-829. 10.1016/j.surg.2009.11.013.

[26] de Almeida Leite RM, de Souza AV, Bay CP, Cauley C,

Bordeianou L, Goldstone R, et al. Delayed operative Management in Complicated Acute Appendicitis-is Avoiding Extended Resection Worth the wait ? Results from a global cohort study. Journal of Gastrointestinal Surgery 2022;**26**:1482-1489. 10.1007/s11605-022-05311-2

[27] Fugazzola P, Coccolini F, Tomasoni M, Stella M, Ansaloni L. Early appendectomy vs. conservative management in complicated acute appendicitis in children: A meta-analysis. Journal of Pediatric Surgery 2019;**54**:2234-2241. 10.1016/j.jpedsurg.2019.01.065

[28] Vaos G, Dimopoulou A, Gkioka E, Zavras N. Immediate surgery or conservative treatment for complicated acute appendicitis in children? A meta-analysis Journal of Pediatric Surgery 2019;**54**:1365-1371. 10.1016/j.jpedsurg.2018.07.017

[29] Writing Group for the CODA Collaborative, Monsell SE, Voldal EC, Davidson GH, Fischkoff K, Coleman N, et al. Patient factors associated with appendectomy within 30 days of initiating antibiotic treatment for appendicitis. JAMA Surgery 2022;**157**:e216900. 10.1001/jamasurg.2021.6900

[30] Khan MS, Siddiqui MTH, Shahzad N, Haider A, Chaudhry MBH, Alvi R. Factors associated with complicated appendicitis: View from a low-middle income country. Cureus 2019;**11**:e4765. 10.7759/cureus.4765

[31] Wang Y, Sun C-Y, Liu J, Chen Y, Bhan C, Tuason JPW, et al. Is endoscopic retrograde appendicitis therapy a better modality for acute uncomplicated appendicitis? A systematic review and meta-analysis. World Journal of Clinical Cases 2021;**9**:10208-10221. 10.12998/wjcc.v9.i33.10208.

[32] Ding W, Du Z, Zhou X. Endoscopic retrograde appendicitis therapy for management of acute appendicitis. Surgical Endoscopy 2022;**36**:2480-2487. 10.1007/s00464-021-08533-8

[33] Ashbrook M, Cheng V, Sandhu K, Matsuo K, Schellenberg M, Inaba K, et al. Management of Complicated Appendicitis during Pregnancy in the US. JAMA Network Open 2022;5:e227555. 10.1001/jamanetworkopen.2022.7555

[34] Lloyd AJ, Abd Elwahab SM, Boland MR, Elfadul A, Hill ADK, Power C. Acute complicated appendicitis caused by an ingested toothpick - A case report. International Journal of Surgery Case Reports 2022;**92**:106872. 10.1016/j.ijscr.2022.106872

[35] Mekakas A, Nagorni E-A, Tablaridis T. Complicated appendicitis: A surgical controversy concerning risk factors, diagnostic algorithm and therapeutic management. Doubts, Problems and Certainties about Acute Appendicitis 2022. 10.5772/intechopen.97270

[36] Neogi S, Banerjee A, Panda SS, Ratan SK, Narang R. Laparoscopic versus open appendicectomy for complicated appendicitis in children: A systematic review and meta-analysis. Journal of Pediatric Surgery 2022;**57**:394-405. 10.1016/j.jpedsurg.2021.07.005

[37] Oh YJ, Sung NS, Choi WJ, Yoon DS, Choi IS, Lee SE, et al. Single incision laparoscopic appendectomy for management of complicated appendicitis: Comparison between single-incision and conventional. Journal of Minimum Invasive Surgery 2018;**21**:148-153. 10.7602/jmis.2018.21.4.148

[38] Foster D, Kethman W, Cai LZ, Weiser TG, Forrester JD. Surgical site

infections after appendectomy performed in low and middle human development-index countries: A systematic review. Surgical Infections 2018;**19**:237-244. 10.1089/sur.2017.188

[39] Sun F, Wang H, Zhang F, Zhang X, Xing Z, Zhang S, et al. Copious irrigation versus suction alone during laparoscopic appendectomy for complicated appendicitis in adults. Journal of Investigative Surgery 2018;**31**:342-346. 10.1080/08941939.2017.1319995

[40] Siotos C, Stergios K, Prasath V, Seal SM, Duncan MD, Sakran JV, et al. Irrigation versus suction in laparoscopic appendectomy for complicated appendicitis: A Meta-analysis. The Journal of Surgical Research 2019;**235**:237-243. 10.1016/j.jss.2018.10.005

[41] Fujishiro J, Fujiogi M, Hirahara N, Terui K, Okamoto T, Watanabe E, et al. Abdominal drainage at appendectomy for complicated appendicitis in children: A propensity-matched comparative study. Annals of Surgery 2021;274:e599–e604. 10.1097/SLA.0000000000003804

[42] Abu A, Mohamedahmed AY, Alamin A, Mohamed M, Osman M, Mohammed MJ, et al. Evaluation of drain insertion after Appendicectomy for complicated appendicitis: A systematic review and Meta-analysis. Cureus 2022;**14**:e32018. 10.7759/cureus.32018

[43] van den Boom AL, de Wijkerslooth EML, Wijnhoven BPL. Systematic review and Meta-analysis of postoperative antibiotics for patients with a complex appendicitis. Digestive Surgery 2020;**37**:101-110. 10.1159/000497482

[44] Panshin MS, Alnachoukati OK, Schroeppel TJ, Metzler M, McFann K, Dunn JA. Optimal duration of antibiotics following appendectomy for patients with complicated appendicitis. The American Surgeon 2021;**87**:480-485. 10.1177/0003134820947372

[45] Ramson DM, Gao H, Penny-Dimri JC, Liu Z, Khong JN, Caruana CB, et al. Duration of post-operative antibiotic treatment in acute complicated appendicitis: Systematic review and meta-analysis. ANZ Journal of Surgery 2021;**91**:1397-1404. 10.1111/ans.16615

[46] Ketha B, Stephenson KJ, Dassinger MS 3rd, Smith SD, Burford JM. Eliminating use of home Oral antibiotics in Pediatric complicated appendicitis. The Journal of Surgical Research 2021;**263**:151-154. 10.1016/j.jss.2020.12.059

[47] Andrey V, Crisinel P-A, Prodhom G, Croxatto A, Joseph J-M. Impact of co-amoxicillin-resistant Escherichia coli and Pseudomonas aeruginosa on the rate of infectious complications in paediatric complicated appendicitis. Swiss Medical Weekly 2019;**149**:w20055. 10.4414/smw.2019.20055

[48] Son JT, Lee GC, Kim HO, Kim T, Lee D, Lee SR, et al. Routine intraoperative bacterial culture may Be needed in complicated appendicitis. Annals of Coloproctology 2020;**36**:155-162. 10.3393/ac.2019.11.04.1

[49] Kwok CPD, Tsui SYB, Chan KWE. Updates on bacterial resistance and empirical antibiotics treatment of complicated acute appendicitis in children. Journal of Pediatric Surgery 2021;**56**:1145-1149. 10.1016/j.jpedsurg.2021.03.027

[50] van Coller R, Arnold M, le Roux H, Tootla H, Dix-Peek S, Nuttal J, et al. Amoxycillin/clavulanic acid monotherapy in complicated

paediatric appendicitis: Good enough? Journal of Pediatric Surgery 2022;**57**:1115-1118. 10.1016/j.jpedsurg.2022.01.032

[51] Aravind, Varkey S, Binu. Post-operative complications of complicated paediatric appendicitis in a tertiary teaching hospital. International Journal of Research Review in Applied Science 2022;**9**:9-16 10.52403/ijrr.20220102

[52] Yamada T, Endo H, Hasegawa H, Kimura T, Kakeji Y, Koda K, et al. Risk of emergency surgery for complicated appendicitis: Japanese nationwide study. Annals of Gastroenterological Surgery. 2021;**5**:236-242. DOI: 10.1002/ags3.12408

Chapter 8

Laparoscopic versus Open Surgery for Suspected Appendicitis

Mohamed Mahmoud Eltaweel

Abstract

Laparoscopic appendectomy has mostly replaced open surgery. Appendectomy is one of the most common operations. This study compared laparoscopic and open surgery for suspected appendicitis. A total of 200 individuals with probable appendicitis participated in this prospective randomized clinical study. All patients over the age of 18 who had a clinical diagnosis of appendicitis were randomly randomized to either open appendectomy (OA) or laparoscopic appendectomy (LA). First prophylactic antimicrobial treatment was administered intravenously. Supine posture and general anesthesia were provided to all patients. After the operation, we followed up for complications and survival. The operating time in laparoscopic patients was significantly greater. However, blood loss was substantially lower. The need for analgesics was substantially reduced in the laparoscopic group. There was a substantial difference between included patients in both groups in terms of postoperative stay length, time to return to work/normal activities, and the incidence of postoperative complications. In terms of survival time or complication incidence, there was no significant difference between the two groups. Despite the longer operational time, LA has a favorable hands-on OA in terms of blood loss, length of postoperative stay, time to return to work/normal activities.

Keywords: appendectomy, appendicitis, laparoscopic, open surgery

1. Introduction

In Egypt, the majority of persons with stomach pain seek medical assistance in emergency rooms each year [1]. The underlying causes of pain range from benign processes to potentially fatal disorders. The prompt diagnosis and treatment of conditions for which a delay in care might have significant consequences remain a problem. The most common emergency abdominal surgery is an appendectomy [2].

Although appendicitis is commonly diagnosed in young boys with stomach pain, the diagnostic variables for premenopausal women with a comparable clinical presentation are more difficult [3]. Furthermore, stomach pain in the elderly might be difficult to diagnose owing to delays in seeking medical attention or difficulty compiling a history and performing a thorough physical examination [4]. Because delayed diagnosis and treatment of appendicitis are associated with a higher risk of perforation, which leads to increased morbidity and mortality, quick intervention is crucial [5].

Although laparoscopy has been promoted for appendicitis diagnosis, its invasiveness has precluded it from being extensively employed. Minimally invasive abdominal surgery became extensively employed in a very short time with the introduction of laparoscopic appendicectomy [6]. Laparoscopic appendicectomy was not previously used to treat acute appendicitis since open appendicectomy had fewer risks and side effects. It is, however, now routinely used in hospitals and has been demonstrated to be a safe therapy [7].

Laparoscopic appendectomy has mainly taken the place of open surgery. Appendectomy, or surgical removal of the appendix, is one of the most common procedures done by a specialized surgeon and is used to teach the foundations of laparoscopy - first by watching and then autonomously conducting the procedure. Preoperative preparation, accurate diagnosis, good surgical technique, and follow-up treatment are the foundations of successful care. The anatomy of the patient must be considered while placing trocars [8].

The appendix is usually straightforward to locate, however, its position and location may fluctuate. The appendix's base and artery are ligated during the treatment, and the appendix is removed in a plastic bag [9]. A healthy appendix should also be removed, although in this case, other causes of the symptoms should be examined. A burst appendix requires significantly more difficult surgical excision, and peritonitis should be treated as quickly as feasible [10]. A periappendicular abscess is a difficult procedure that should be conducted during the day. Most people who have undergone a non-perforated appendix ectomy may go home within 23 hours after the operation [11].

In this study, we compared laparoscopic and open surgery for suspected appendicitis.

2. Material and methods

A total of 200 individuals with probable appendicitis participated in this prospective randomized clinical study. The study was performed in Al Azhar University Hospitals from December 2018 to February 2021. All patients over the age of 18 who had a clinical diagnosis of appendicitis were randomly chosen for either open appendectomy (OA) or laparoscopic appendectomy (LA).

Exclusion criteria: Patients who had prior abdominal surgery or anesthesia reasons that made laparoscopy impossible. Another significant pathology that would change surgical therapy was found in patients who agreed to appendicectomy.

3. Methods

Prophylactic antimicrobial treatment was administered intravenously (IV) during anesthesia induction, including 1 g of Cefoxitin and 500mg of Metronidazole. Antibiotics were supplied for 48 hours if there was an appendiceal perforation or peritoneal abscess. Using a typical right iliac fossa incision and gridiron technique, two consultant surgeons and one surgical registrar conducted an open appendicectomy. As is typical, the appendix was removed, and the incision was healed in layers. A subcuticular 3/0 proline suture was used to keep the skin closed. There were no drains created.

One experienced consultant surgeon and a surgical registrar executed the laparoscopic appendicectomy under the instruction of the others. The gadget was fully non-disposable. Supine posture and general anesthesia were provided to the patient. A catheter was inserted in the urinary system if the patient could not pee promptly before the procedure. A 10 mm cannula was placed just below the umbilicus and a pneumoperitoneum was generated before introducing the laparoscope into the peritoneal cavity.

A comprehensive examination of the abdominal organs was done. The laparoscopic examination might reveal the presence or absence of the appendix. The surgical table was adjusted head-down and left side down to reposition the small intestine away from the pelvic and right iliac fossa (RIF). At McBurney's site, a 5 mm cannula was placed under strict monitoring. Fluid was aspirated from the pelvic organs after they had been properly evaluated. A 10 mm cannula was inserted under direct vision into the iliac fossa on the left side of the body. There could be no activity without utilizing this port. Using atraumatic grasping forceps, the appendix was grabbed and lifted cephalad through the 5 mm incision. If the appendix was thickened, a catgut endloop was introduced at the tip to facilitate retraction and remove the need for gripping forceps. If the appendix was retrocaecal, the caecum and ascending colon were mobilized using laparoscopic scissor dissection. To locate the mesoappendix, doctors used non-disposable laparoscopic clip applicators. Once the mesoappendix was located, it was cut and coagulated close to the appendix. Chromic catgut endoloop was employed to hold the appendix in place. After then, it was taken out. A distal clip was utilized to release the appendix from the ligature. To avoid damaging the skin or subcutaneous tissues, the appendix was retrieved using a 10 mm LIF cannula.

A large forceps was used to widen the port hole and remove the appendix if it became too thick to be drawn through the cannula. The wound was then irrigated with 10% povidone-iodine and any purulent fluid in the peritoneal cavity was suctioned out and saline lavaged. The wounds were closed with Dexon sutures and no drains were constructed.

To objectively evaluate discomfort, the number of narcotic injections or oral analgesics required to manage postoperative pain was employed. There were several post-operative problems. Wound infection was defined as one that required drainage or treatment for erythema in duration or pus. The duration of the postoperative stay was recorded, with day 1 being the day of surgery. Patients were freed if they were able to eat a normal meal and showed symptoms of propulsive bowel function (i.e. flatus, bowel action) (i.e. flatus, bowel action).

Following that, the patient had an outpatient examination or a direct phone conversation concerning their return to work, sports, or normal activities. Patients were given a certificate of sickness that was valid until their next outpatient appointment. All patients were assessed in the outpatient clinic for postoperative complications between the seventh and tenth postoperative days.

Based on specific histological findings, one pathologist evaluated the histology and rated the severity of appendicitis (**Table 1**).

Normal appendix	No mucosal abnormality
Mild acute appendicitis	Mucosal ulceration and/or intraluminal pus
Suppurative	Transmural inflammation appendicitis
Gangrenous appendicitis	Cellular necrosis with or without perforation

Table 1.
Histological grades of appendicitis.

4. Ethical considerations

The study was approved by the Ethics Board of Al-Azhar University and informed written consent was taken from each participant in the study. All the patients were informed about the surgery and the autotransplantation technique, value, and possible complications. This work has been carried out following The Code of Ethics of the World Medical Association (Declaration of Helsinki) for studies involving humans.

Statistical Analysis: IBM SPSS version 22.0 was used to analyze computer-generated data. To express quantitative data, percentages and numbers were employed. Before utilizing the median in nonparametric analysis or the interquartile range in parametric analysis, it was required to perform Kolmogorov-Smirnov tests to ensure that the data were normal. We used the (0.05) significance threshold to establish the significance of the findings. The Chi-Square test is used to compare two or more groups. The Monte Carlo test may be used to adjust for any number of cells with a count less than 5. Fischer Chi-Square adjustment was applied to tables demonstrating non-continuous data.

5. Results

In terms of basal features, there was no significant difference between included patients in both groups (**Table 2**).

There was no significant difference in the distribution of appendicitis macroscopically or histologically between the enrolled participants in both groups (**Table 3**).

There was a nonsignificant difference between included subjects regarding ASA grade. Operative time was significantly longer in laparoscopic cases ($P < 0.001$). However, blood loss was significantly decreased in this group compared with the open surgery group. Also, the need for analgesics was significantly lower in the laparoscopic group (**Table 4**).

	Laparoscopic (N = 100)	Open surgery (N = 100)	P-Value
Age	45.5 ± 12.3	43.7 ± 11.8	0.29
Sex			
Male	55 (55%)	62 (62%)	0.32
Female	45 (45%)	38 (38%)	
BMI (kg/m^2)	23.65 ± 4.5	24.1 ± 3.2	0.42
Co-morbidities			
HTN	14 (14%)	13 (13%)	0.81
DM	11 (11%)	10 (10%)	
Other	5 (5%)	7 (7%)	
Time from diagnosis to surgery (Hours)	25.01 ± 11.54	27.51 ± 13.02	0.15
Previous abdominal surgery	19 (19%)	26 (26%)	0.24
WBC >10.000/ml	70 (70%)	67 (67%)	0.65
Preoperative CRP (mg/dL)	13.26 ± 7.5	14.63 ± 8.3	0.37

Table 2.
Patients' basal characteristics.

	Laparoscopic (N = 100)	Open surgery (N = 100)	P-Value
Macroscopically inflamed appendix	41 (41%)	53 (53%)	0.089
Histological appendicitis	41 (41%)	53 (53%)	0.089
Macroscopically normal appendix	58 (58%)	47 (47%)	0.12
Histological appendicitis	12 (12%)	10 (10%)	0.65

Table 3.
Appendix specimens macroscopic vs microscopic findings in open versus laparoscopic appendicectomy.

	Laparoscopic (N = 100)	Open surgery (N = 100)	P-Value
ASA grade			
I	70 (70%)	65 (65%)	0.73
II	18 (18%)	22 (22%)	
III	12 (12%)	13 (13%)	
Operative time (min)	89.26 ± 32.48	68.25 ± 18.36	0.0001
Blood loss (g)	38.62 ± 12.69	86.5 ± 20.15	0.0001
Need for analgesics	18 (18%)	32 (32%)	0.022

Table 4.
Operation characteristics.

	Laparoscopic (N = 100)	Open surgery (N = 100)	P-Value
Days to resumption of liquids	1.3 ± 0.44	1.4 ± 0.42	0.1
Days to resumption of solids	4.3 ± 2.1	4.8 ± 2.2	0.1
Days to walking	1.6 ± 0.71	1.7 ± 0.62	0.29
Duration of drainage (days)	5.2 ± 6.7	5.9 ± 7.3	0.48
Duration of intravenous antibiotics (days)	5.6 ± 3.3	4.8 ± 2.7	0.62
Length of postoperative stay (days)	6.7 ± 2.3	7.7 ± 2.5	0.0036
Time taken to return to work/ normal activities (days)	9.5 ± 4.3	11.4 ± 3.6	0.0001
Post-operative complications occurrence			
SSI	6 (6%)	18 (18%)	0.009
Leakage	3 (3%)	7 (7%)	0.19
Bowel obstruction	4 (4%)	3 (3%)	0.7
Other	5 (5%)	10 (10%)	0.18
Total	18 (18%)	38 (38%)	0.0016

Table 5.
Post-operative follow-up outcomes.

There was a substantial difference between included participants in both groups in terms of postoperative stay length, time to return to work/normal activities, and the incidence of postoperative problems. All were decreased in the LA group. Regarding Post operative complications occurrence SSI was significantly more observable in the open surgery group (**Table 5**).

There was a significant correlation between open surgery and complications occurrence (**Table 6**).

There was no significant difference between the two groups regarding survival time and complication occurrence (**Figure 1** and **Table 7**).

		Complication
Surgery	Pearson Correlation	0.223**
	P-Value	0.002

Table 6.
Correlation between surgery and occurred complications.

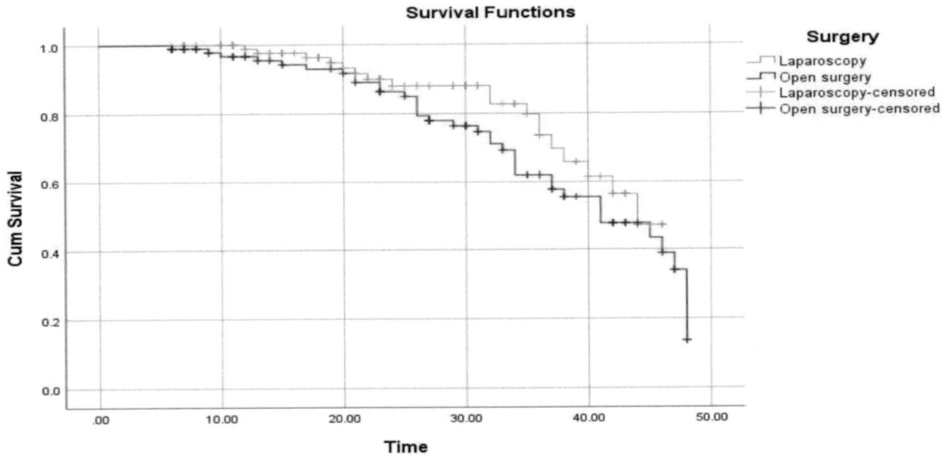

Figure 1.
Survival correlation between surgery and time between diagnosis and surgery.

Surgery	Mean[a]				Median			
	Estimate	Std. error	95% confidence interval		Estimate	Std. error	95% Confidence interval	
			Lower bound	Upper bound			Lower bound	Upper bound
Laparoscopic	39.790	1.220	37.398	42.182	44.000			
Open Surgery	37.920	1.358	35.259	40.581	41.000	4.006	33.147	48.853
Overall	39.135	.966	37.240	41.029	44.000	2.111	39.862	48.138
Overall comparisons								
			Chi-square				P-value	
Log Rank (Mantel-Cox)			1.632				.201	

Table 7.
Survival correlation between surgery and time between diagnosis and surgery.

6. Discussion

Acute appendicitis in particular is a potentially fatal condition. Although surgical appendicitis was described in the eighteenth century, appendicitis' therapeutic implications were not recognized until the late nineteenth century [12]. With the development of improved anesthetics and antibiotics, OA has emerged as the gold standard for treating acute appendicitis. There are dangers associated with open appendicectomy, such as wound infection rates exceeding 5% and postoperative adhesions that cause small intestinal blockage [13]. In addition, despite advancements in ultrasonography and computer-aided diagnosis, a considerable number of normal appendicectomy cases are still being done. Misdiagnosis is especially common in women, with appendicectomy rates ranging from 20 to 47 percent [14].

The efficacy of the laparoscopic method for appendicitis has been well researched. However, because of a paucity of high-level data, the relevance of laparoscopy in appendicitis remains unknown (e.g., randomized controlled trials). The current randomized controlled study investigated whether LA for appendicitis successfully lowers the frequency of postoperative complications and improves several postoperative recovery parameters in adults when compared to OA. In our investigation, there was no significant variation in basic features between included patients in both groups.

In our research, there was a considerable increase in the amount of time spent on patients treated with LA. This has been documented in several earlier investigations, such as Taguchi et al. Blood loss was much reduced in the LA group in our investigation, which is consistent with Shimoda et al. results. Another difficulty in the comparison of LA and OA is the longer operational duration and substantial blood loss during LA. In general, those two parameters are determined by the surgeon's expertise [15]. Although the majority of surgical staff have done basic and advanced laparoscopic operations, operating time is considerable when performed by novice surgeons and is reduced by gaining knowledge. Blood loss is also affected by the surgeon's expertise and the severity of appendicitis. In our research, the quantity of blood lost during the LA technique was much reduced.

Shortening postoperative hospital stay is one of the most essential criteria for a medical institution's economic management, and to shorten postoperative hospital stay, surgeons must limit the risk of postoperative complications to the best of their abilities. SSI is the most significant postoperative complication in terms of prolonging stay for patients after appendectomy. In our research, there was a significant difference between included participants in both groups in terms of postoperative stay length, time to return to work/normal activities, and the incidence of postoperative problems. Shimoda et al. also found that all were reduced in the LA group. In terms of post-operative complications, SSI was substantially more common in the open surgery group.

According to a recent meta-analysis [16], the overall incidence of SSI varies from 0 to 37.4 per 100 appendectomies (95% CI: 1.0–17.6). The incidence ranged from 5.8 per 100 appendectomies in Europe to 12.6 per 100 in Africa, according to a subgroup study that looked at the causes of variation (p less than 0.0001). SSI following appendectomy rose with decreasing wealth, from 6.2 per 100 appendectomies in high-income countries to 11.1 per 100 appendectomies in low-income countries ($p = 0.015$). Open appendectomy (11.0 per 100 surgical procedures) had a greater incidence of SSI ($p = 0.0002$) than laparoscopic (4.6 per 100 appendectomies).

Taguchi et al. found no statistically significant difference between OA and LA in terms of post- operative hospital stay or liquids and solids resumption. Older research [17] found a substantial difference between the OA and LA groups when it came to resuming normal activities.

The possibility cannot be ruled out that analgesic treatment might not always accurately represent actual pain levels, since this may be dictated by department norms or standards rather than actual demand. To measure postoperative pain, a visual analog scale may be more suitable. It is possible that the advantages of LA would become more apparent in more difficult situations [18], or that there would be some changes in the severity of sicknesses, such as inflammatory response, discomfort, expense, and time of healing, between small and big infected incisions.

There was a strong association between OA and the development of complications in our research. We also discovered no statistically significant difference between the two groups in terms of survival time and complication incidence. So, in spite of urgent situations, time spent on stabilization and preparation for surgery is vital, with no substantial increase in the probability of complication incidence after each operation.

7. Conclusion

Despite the lengthier operating time, LA has a superior hands-on OA in terms of blood loss, postoperative stay duration, time to return to work/normal activities, and postoperative problems. In terms of survival time or complication incidence, there was no significant difference between the two groups.

Funding

No fund.

Conflicts of interest

The authors declare no conflicts of interest regarding the publication of this paper.

Available competing interests

None.

Consent for publication

I confirm that all authors accept the manuscript for submission

Author details

Mohamed Mahmoud Eltaweel
Faculty of Medicine, General Surgery Department, Al Azhar University, Cairo, Egypt

*Address all correspondence to: dr.mo1718@gmail.com

References

[1] Mohey A. Primary healthcare emergency services in Alexandria, Egypt 2016. Quality in Primary Care. 2017;**25**(5):303

[2] Zachariah S, Fenn M, Jacob K, et al. Management of acute abdomen in pregnancy: Current perspectives. International Journal of Women's Health. 2019;**11**:119

[3] Yang H, Wang R, Zhao L, et al. Diagnosis and analysis of transabdominal and intracavitary ultrasound in gynecological acute abdomen. Computational and Mathematical Methods in Medicine. 29 Dec 2021. DOI: 10.1155/2021/9508838

[4] Bhangu A. Evaluation of appendicitis risk prediction models in adults with suspected appendicitis. 2020

[5] Snyder M, Guthrie M, Cagle D. Acute appendicitis: Efficient diagnosis and management. American Family Physician. 2018;**98**(1):25-33

[6] Virdis F, Podda M, Reccia I, et al. Laparoscopy and minimally invasive surgery techniques in acute care surgery. In: Chiara O, editors. Trauma Centers and Acute Care Surgery. Updates in Surgery. Springer, Cham; 2022. DOI: 10.1007/978-3-030-73155-7_19

[7] Barie P. Non-operative management of appendicitis: Evolution, not revolution. Surgical Infections. 2021;**22**(10):991-1003

[8] Walędziak M, Lasek A, Wysocki M, et al. Risk factors for serious morbidity, prolonged length of stay, and hospital readmission after laparoscopic appendectomy-results from Pol-LA (Polish Laparoscopic Appendectomy) multicenter large cohort study. Scientific Reports. 2019;**9**(1):1-9

[9] Ismail Z, Mohamed M, Rizk A, et al. Laparoscopic appendectomy for perforated appendicitis; a comparison with open appendectomy. SVU-International Journal of Medical Sciences. 2020;**3**(2):69-78

[10] Petroianu A. Relevant aspects of acute appendicitis. Revista da Associação Médica Brasileira. 2022;**68**:121-124

[11] Nechay T, Sazhin A, Titkova S, et al. Evaluation of enhanced recovery after surgery program components implemented in laparoscopic appendectomy: A prospective randomized clinical study. Scientific Reports. 2020;**10**(1):1-8

[12] Young P. Appendicitis and its history. Revista Médica de Chile. 2014;**142**(**5**): 667-672

[13] Pokala N, Sadhasivam S, Kiran R, et al. Complicated appendicitis-is the laparoscopic approach appropriate? A comparative study with the open approach: Outcome in a community hospital setting. The American Surgeon. 2007;**73**(8):737-742

[14] Pradhan S, Shakya Y, Batajoo H, et al. Laparoscopic versus open appendectomy: A prospective comparative study. Journal of Society of Surgeons of Nepal. 2015;**18**(2):29-32

[15] Shimoda M, Maruyama T, Nishida K, et al. Preoperative high C-reactive protein level is associated with an increased likelihood for conversion from laparoscopic to open appendectomy in

patients with acute appendicitis. Clinical and Experimental Gastroenterology. 2019;**12**:141

[16] Danwang C, Bigna J, Tochie J, et al. Global incidence of surgical site infection after appendectomy: A systematic review and meta-analysis. BMJ Open. 2020;**10**(2):e034266

[17] Kollias J, Harries R, Otto G, et al. Laparoscopic versus open appendicectomy for suspected appendicitis: A prospective study. Australian and New Zealand Journal of Surgery. 1994;**64**(12):830-835

[18] Horvath P, Lange J, Bachmann R, et al. Comparison of clinical outcome of laparoscopic versus open appendectomy for complicated appendicitis. Surgical Endoscopy. 2017;**31**(1):199-205

Section 3

Current Treatments and Nursing Management of Appendicitis

Chapter 9

Current Treatments for Appendicitis

Abdulrahman Alotaibi

Abstract

One out of every 1000 persons is diagnosed with acute appendicitis (AA) each year. Men are slightly more likely to have AA than women (8.6% vs. 6.7%). A simple or uncomplicated appendicitis is one that is characterized by inflammation and fluid around the appendix. It is recommended that patients with AA undergo a history and physical examination, with attention paid to temperature and rebound tenderness, followed by laboratory tests and radiology studies. A number of indices have been investigated in order to improve the accuracy of diagnosis. CT's diagnostic sensitivity and specificity are not significantly different whether contrast-enhanced or nonenhanced CT is utilized to diagnose the patient. Numerous studies have proved the safety and effectiveness of laparoscopic appendectomy (LA) for adults. There is mounting evidence that noninvasive therapies, such as those that focus on pain management and draining collection, maybe just as effective as surgery for uncomplicated appendicitis.

Keywords: acute appendicitis, complicated appendicitis, laparoscopic appendectomy, appendectomy, nonoperative management, hospital length of stay LOS

1. Introduction

Approximately one out of every 1000 persons are diagnosed with acute appendicitis (AA) each year [1]. While men are slightly more likely to have AA than women (8.6% vs. 6.7%), women are more likely to undergo an appendectomy (23.1% vs. 12.0%) [2]. According to its severity, AA is either classified as "uncomplicated" or "complicated" by the European Association of Endoscopic Surgery (EAES) [3]. A simple or uncomplicated appendicitis is one that is characterized by inflammation and a small amount of fluid or an abscess around the appendix. An abscess collection, phlegmon mass, gangrene, perforation, or peritonitis are present in cases of complex appendicitis (CA). Phlegmons are inflammatory benign mass or tumors composed of appendices, their adjoining viscera, and the omentum (**Table 1**) [1, 4].

It is recommended that patients with AA undergo a history and physical examination, with attention paid to temperature and rebound tenderness, followed by laboratory tests and radiology studies. The results of a pregnancy test should be obtained by all women of childbearing age. It is important to note that the clinical presentation of AA varies even within the same age group. For instance, among children younger than 5 years of age, the presentation is more complicated due to rapid progression and

	Uncomplicated	Complicated
Criteria		
Inflammation	+	+
Gangrene	–	+
Phlegmon	–	+
Perityphlitic abscess	–	+
Free fluid	–	+
Perforation	–	+

Table 1.
Criteria for distinguishing between uncomplicated vs. complicated appendicitis, based on the European Association of Endoscopic Surgery (EAES), 2016.

perforation. A comparative study of 142 children found that children less than 5years of age have a 44% chance of developing perforated appendicitis with abscess, while children between 5 and 10 years of age have a 13% chance, p = 0.001 [5].

2. Challenges in the diagnosis

It is a dilemma if appendicitis is not diagnosed in a timely manner, as it can result in perforation of adverse consequences. A perforation can be sealed with phlegmon or abscesses, or it may be free with septicemia and peritonitis. Additionally, it is possible to operate on a negative appendectomy due to an incorrect diagnosis.

A number of indices have been investigated in order to improve the accuracy of diagnosis. The mean platelet volume (MPV), plateletcrit, and platelet distribution width are some of the recent indices. The diagnosis may be bolstered by elevated levels of leukocytes, inflammatory markers, plateletcrit, [6] and low MPV according to one systematic review [7].

To support their clinical judgment, most clinicians use certain scores in addition to radiology scans. The modified Alvarado Score and the Appendicitis Inflammatory Response Score (AIRS) are the most commonly utilized scores in clinical settings (**Table 2**) [1, 8, 9].

In cases when the likelihood is unsure or intermediate, the score is backed up by several scan modalities. For children and thin patients, ultrasonography (US) is the method of choice, while pregnant women are advised to have a magnetic resonance image (MRI) [10]. When it comes to women of childbearing age, the morbidly obese, and the elderly, computed tomography (CT) is the gold standard for diagnosing appendicitis.

CT's diagnostic sensitivity and specificity are not significantly different whether contrast-enhanced or nonenhanced CT is utilized to diagnose the patient. One study examined the performance of CT scans with and without contrast on 140 patients, and the accuracy remained between 80 and 87% without statistically significant differences [11]. That finding is vital, particularly when a patient has a renal impairment and is suspected of having AA. The diameter of the appendix that should be considered too small to be indicative of AA varies. Some have proposed a CT scan threshold of 9.25 mm for making the diagnosis [11].

Criterion		Alvarado score	AIR score
Symptoms			
Vomiting		—	1
Nausea or vomiting		1	—
Anorexia		1	—
RLQ pain		2	1
Migratory RLQ pain		1	—
Signs			
RLQ rebound pain or guarding		1	—
	mild	—	1
	moderate	—	2
	severe	—	3
Body temperature	>37.5 °C	1	—
	>38.5°C	—	1
Laboratory parameters			
Leukocyte count	>10,000/L	2	—
	10,000–14,900/L	—	1
	>15,000/L	—	2
Leukocyte shift		1	—
PMN granulocytes	70–84%	—	1
	≥ 85%	—	2
CRP value	10–49 mg/L	—	1
	≥ 50 mg/L	—	2
Sum		10	12
Alvarado score		<5	low probability
		5–6	unclear
		7–8	likely
		>8	high probability
AIR score		<5	low probability
		5–8	intermediate probability
		>8	high probability

AIR: Appendicitis Inflammatory Response; RLQ: right lower abdominal quadrant; PMN: polymorphonuclear; and CRP: C-reactive protein.

Table 2.
Modified Alvarado and AIR scores.

It is not always possible to tell the difference between simple and severe appendicitis using ultrasound, CT, or MR. Even though CT's sensitivity is low, it has a significant negative predictive value for CA [12].

As opposed to the intraoperative finding, CT scans are not as effective in detecting perforations. In one study, 89 individuals presenting with right lower quadrant discomfort underwent CT imaging and appendectomy.

The pathology results reveal that perforation had occurred in 48% (43/89), 93% (n = 40) of perforations were overlooked by radiography [13].

According to the results of a single systematic review and meta-analysis of CT Features for differentiating complicated and uncomplicated appendicitis. This research identifies 10 useful CT characteristics for distinguishing CA [14]. The overall pooled specificity for the presence of an extra or intraluminal appendicolith, abscess, wall-enhancing defect, extra or intraluminal air, ileus, periappendiceal fluid collection, or ascites was more than 70%. Only stranding of fat around the appendix was very sensitive 94%. in addition to the aforementioned, one of the most sensitive and specific sonographic findings for differentiating complex from uncomplicated appendicitis was the absence of the typically echogenic submucosal layer (sensitivity 100% and specificity 92%) [15].

3. Surgical management and outcome

Numerous studies have proved the safety and effectiveness of laparoscopic appendectomy (LA) for adults. A total of 1251 LA and 898 open appendectomies (OA) were compared in one meta-analysis consisting of 16 researches, 9 of which were randomized controlled trials [16]. Reduced inflammation, quicker recovery and hospital time, earlier bowel function restoration, and shorter operation times are all advantages of laparoscopic over conventional surgery. This is due to the fact that less tissue damage occurs with LA as opposed to open surgery. Although the surgical cost of LA is higher than that of OA, the shorter hospital stay associated with LA makes the total spent for both operations somewhat comparable [17].

Nearly a quarter of surgeons may choose open surgeries on patients less than 18 years old. One review comparing OA with LA in 390 patients (younger than 18 years) found that the minimally invasive technique is linked to less problems and 1 day shorter hospitalization [18].

A debate between surgeons about whether or not it is safe to perform LA on patients with complex conditions. Morbidity, mortality, and duration of hospital stay were significantly reduced in an analysis of 6428 patients with CA, of whom 3174 were treated laparoscopically [19]. This demonstrates not just the safety of LA but also improved recovery and results.

Most patients are subjectively given a diagnosis of CA after surgery; however, there is no consensus on particular intraoperative diagnostic criteria, which may lead to erroneous classification [20]. In one review, including 1066 appendectomies, 239 of them were complicated. Histopathological CA may be predicted by a number of factors, including but not limited to age, elevated heart rate, pain duration, appendix size, and appendicolith presence [20]. Forty percent of patients were misclassified as a result of the surgeon's evaluation. Where there is room for advancement and a better-measured system [20].

Concerns were raised regarding the expense and time commitment involved in sending regular appendix specimens for histopathology. The importance of routine histological testing was the subject of a meta-analysis that comprised 25 studies and 57,357 patients [21].

In 10.6% of cases, the appendix seemed normal, in 88.6% of cases inflammation was present, and in 2.52% of cases abnormalities were discovered (2718 patients). The most common abnormalities were parasitic infections (0.54%), endometriosis (0.03%), granulomatous illness (0.26%), and neoplasms (0.71%). Most neoplasms were neuroendocrine tumors, then adenocarcinoma, and finally lymphoma. The ability of the surgeon in the detection of aberrant appendix at a macroscopic level that necessitates subsequent treatment makes the selective histopathology assessment a potential method. There is currently no agreement on a protocol regarding the use of selective histopathology, which necessitates a precise intraoperative evaluation by the surgeon. To aid surgeons in the detection of aberrant pathology and the minimization of needless histopathology investigation, the FANCY trial is now conducting a cost-benefit analysis of selective histological examination after appendicectomy and cholecystectomy [22].

Surgeons argued for a long time regarding the postoperative abscess after LA. After pooling the results of ten meta-analyses to investigate the post-LA surgical site infection (SSI) and abdominal collection. They discovered that the risk of SSI was about 60% lower in LA than in open surgery, but the rate of the abdominal abscess was twice as high [23]. Contrary to earlier reviews, some did not find any significant difference in the incidence of abdominal abscess with 6.1% in LA group versus 4.6% in OA group, $p = 0.91$ [19].

This forces many surgeons to go outside the box by resorting to techniques like single-port LA or prophylactic peritoneal lavage in order to minimize postoperative abscess. Lavage does not appear to be more effective than suction in preventing post-operative infections, according to a meta-analysis of eight separate investigations [24].

Moreover, there was no statistically significant difference in the incidence of SSI between the 2749 patients treated with a single port and the 2735 patients treated with traditional LA ($p = 0.98$) [25].

Having a complicated appendectomy might add days to patient hospital stay. Reviewing data from 450 patients, researchers found that longer pain duration (HR = 2.37, 95% C.I = 1.09–5.16, P = .029), longer operative time (HR = 2.09, 95% C.I = 1.04–4.21, P = .038), and CA (HR = 6.61, 95% C.I = 2.67–14.21, P = .001) were all significantly associated with longer hospital stays [26]. When compared to less problematic appendicitis, those that are more complicated are associated with significantly higher rates of morbidity, readmission, and up to a 6-fold increase in hospitalization [26]. The approach may modify the required hospitalization time, LA had a shorter duration of stay than OA did for CA (6.4 days against 8.9 days, $p = 0.02$) [19].

4. Nonoperative management (NOM)

In 1930, Bailey et al. documented rest and fasting as part of the conservative therapy of appendicitis before moving on to a delayed elective appendectomy [27]. Also, in 1956, Coldrey et al. reported that antibiotic treatment was used to successfully treat 471 cases of AA, with a very low death rate (0.2%). Furthermore, only 14.4% of patients had a recurrence [28].

Surgical intervention for CA is not without risks, but there is mounting evidence that noninvasive therapies, such as those that focus on pain management and draining collection, may be just as effective. Téoule P et al. [1], in particular when technical variables, such as the presence of phlegmon or suspicion of malignancy, lead to improper ileocecal resection or right-sided hemicolectomy, as was the case in around 3.4% (17/493) of patients in one study [4, 29].

However, there is currently little data to support the use of conservative therapy for simple cases of appendicitis, making surgery the preferred option for both children and adults [1]. Patients in the 11 trials (5 randomized clinical trials RCTs, 3 retrospective studies, and 3 prospective cohort studies) totaling 2751 were split into two groups: those who received conservative treatment (n = 1463) and those who had surgery (n = 1288) [30]. Conservative treatment resulted in an 83% success rate (95% CI: 77.2–88.2%), a 10.3% incidence of complication (95% CI: 8.5–12.6%), a 5.6% need surgery (95% CI: 3.1–10.2%), and a 0.47 day longer length of stay than the surgical group.

In a meta-analysis, 3618 individuals with uncomplicated appendicitis were assigned to antibiotics (n = 1743) or appendectomy (n = 1875) [31]. There was a failure rate of 8.5% for antibiotic therapy, and a recurrence rate of 19.2% at the 1-year follow-up. The risk of perforation was low, and it was not considerably increased by nonoperative treatment.

While the effectiveness of nonsurgical therapy is quite well, it is somewhat lower than that of appendectomy; nevertheless, the rate of complications is much lower than that of urgent surgery [32, 33].

When it comes to nonsurgical treatments, how long they really work is up for debate. One study found that, among children, 82% of NOM are still effective after 4 years, whereas 14% have seen a recurrence [32]. Another found that the NOM plan using just antibiotics had a 67.1% success rate and was linked to considerably fewer disability days at 1 year compared with urgent surgery [33].

There were 530 participants in the APPAC trial, and they were randomly assigned to get either appendectomy (n = 273) or antibiotic treatment (n = 257). Cumulative incidence of appendicitis relapse was 34, 35, 37, and 39% at 2, 3, 4, and 5 years, respectively. At 5 years, the incidence of complications, such as SSI, incisional hernias, obstruction, and pain, was statistically significantly higher in the surgical group with a rate of 24.4% (95% CI: 19.2–30.3%) (n = 60/246), compared to 6.5% (95% CI: 3.8–10.4%) (n = 16/246) in the antibiotic group, p = 0.001 [34].

Appendectomy is still considered the best option for treating acute uncomplicated appendicitis, according to the European Association for Endoscopic Surgery's (EAES) recommendation. This is backed up by a recent meta-analysis of 3203 patients (1613 received antibiotics versus 1590 appendicectomy) [35]. Treatment at 1 year was successful for 1016 of 1613 patients (63%), revealing that antibiotics were less effective than appendicectomy, as well as, hospital readmissions increased by a factor of six [35].

However, definitive findings about the management of complex appendicitis remain elusive [3]. Conservative therapy of AA is not recommended by the Society of American Gastrointestinal and Endoscopic Surgeons (SAGES) and they lean toward discussing the safety, effectiveness, and appropriateness of LA [36].

Antibiotic treatment regimens and durations favored in different studies were widely reported. Initially, single-agent parenteral antibiotics of amoxicillin-clavulanate, piperacillin-tazobactam, or a carbapenem were employed, as well as combination therapies with a second- or third-generation cephalosporin and metronidazole. After leaving the hospital, patients began taking a combination of fluoroquinolone or a third-generation cephalosporin and metronidazole by mouth. Ten days is the typical length of therapy [37].

The high rates of *Escherichia coli* resistance make amoxicillin-clavulanic acid an unwise choice for treating intraabdominal infections, notwithstanding recommendations. In mild-to-moderate community-acquired infections, broad-spectrum regimens are not recommended until antimicrobial resistance is apparent [38, 39]. Persistent pain or discomfort after 48–72 hours of antibiotics may warrant appendectomy [37].

Nonetheless, there are problems that require fixing with conservative therapy such as the benefits of NOM over appendectomy in cases of microperforation, comorbidities, pediatrics, and geriatrics. Long-term risks of recurrence or undetected cancer. The optimal treatment plan, duration, response criteria, and when appendectomy is needed [37].

5. New practice of colonoscopic drainage

Despite advances in treatment, the appendicular abscess is difficult to manage. For stable patients, radiologically guided drainage is the therapy of choice. There was a 25% failure rate for percutaneous drainage in a study of 2209 appendiceal abscesses, which lead to longer hospital stays and higher overall costs [40].

Lower abscess grade, CT-guided drainage, and a transgluteal route have been linked to a higher incidence of abscess clearance than higher abscess grades, ultrasound-guided drainage, and transabdominal approaches [41].

Some have suggested using colonoscopy and internal drainage of the abscess to promote healing and rule out cancer prior to interval appendectomy, as an alternative to external drainage, which has risks of colocutaneous fistula and a lower chance of success [42].

One of the most cutting-edge techniques is endoscopic retrograde appendicitis treatment (ERAT), which is performed *via* the patient's natural orifice (NOTES) [43]. By combining diagnosis and therapy, we may get a precise picture of what is going on, eliminate other possible causes of colonic symptoms, and get rid of fecal stones and abscesses all at once.

Abscess draining into the cecum is performed after cannulating the appendiceal orifice. Despite that, ERAT is not an option for patients who had a ruptured appendix, periappendiceal abscess, or an allergy to the contrast agent. While the average operating time for ERAT was longer (50 minutes) than that of LA (10–15 minutes), the procedure might prevent surgery, lessen pain and need for antibiotics, and accelerate the return to normal activities [44].

6. Unexpected finding

Surgeons might trouble by unexpected findings on histopathology, such as neuroendocrine tumor (NET) or epithelial neoplasm. When such results are obtained, the surgeon must decide whether or not to do a right hemicolectomy (RHC) with the purpose of removing a sufficient number of lymph nodes or achieving negative margins.

Appendiceal cancer categorization proposed by WHO and the International Society for Peritoneal Surface Oncology(PSOGI), which undergoes regular revisions [45, 46].

Nonneoplastic mucinous lesions (as mucocele), invasive adenocarcinomas, low-grade and high-grade appendiceal mucinous neoplasms (LAMN and HAMN), and goblet cell adenocarcinomas are all examples of epithelial neoplasms. On the other hand, well and poorly-differentiated neuroendocrine carcinomas and mixed neuroendocrine-non-neuroendocrine neoplasms (MiNEN) are examples of neuroendocrine neoplasm. A clinical illness known as "pseudomyxoma peritonei (PMP) is defined by the presence of a mucinous appendiceal lesion in addition to widespread mucinous peritoneal involvement.

Although wide debate on post-appendectomy management of adenocarcinoma, The American Society of Colon and Rectal Surgeons 2019 recommends right hemicolectomy for stage I-III disease [47]. Depending on the specifics of each case, further treatments, such as cytotoxic chemotherapy, biological therapy, cytoreductive surgery, and hot intraperitoneal chemotherapy (HIPEC), may be used.

Appendiceal NET has received increasing attention since 1907, when Oberndoder first coined the name carcinoid [48]. North American Neuroendocrine Tumor Society (NANETS) and European Neuroendocrine Tumor Society (ENETS) recommend that only appendiceal NET >20 mm should be treated with a RHC due to the increased risk of nodal positivity in these tumors [49–51].

However, it may be necessary to focus on tumors that are between 10 and 20 mm in diameter at their base, have a Ki-67 index of more than 3%, and have a lymphovascular invasion.

One study of 261 individuals with appendiceal carcinoid tumors found that basing treatment decisions on tumor location, tumor grade, or mesoappendiceal invasion was not only ineffective but also led to needless hemicolectomy. Lymphovascular invasion may help the surgeon decide what to do next for a patient with a 15 mm tumor [52].

The prognosis of appendiceal NETs is better than those of other midgut NETs. The 5-year relative survival rates for patients with localized, regional, and distant metastatic disease are 94, 84.6, and 33.7%, respectively [48, 52].

Goblet cell adenocarcinoma (GCA, previously named goblet cell carcinoids or adenocarcinoids) is another surprising discovery post appendectomy that exhibits characteristics of both NET and adenocarcinomas. It can be distinguished from NET by its positive staining for periodic acid-Schiff (PAS) antigens. Other markers that distinguish GCA from NET include its greater Ki-67 and expression of carcinoembryonic antigen (CEA) [53].

A poorer prognosis than NETs necessitate treatingv GCA as one would invasive adenocarcinoma [54].

Author details

Abdulrahman Alotaibi
University of Jeddah, Jeddah, Saudi Arabia

*Address all correspondence to: aalotaibi@uj.edu.sa

References

[1] Téoule P, Laffolie J, Rolle U, Reissfelder C. Acute appendicitis in childhood and adulthood. Deutsches Ärzteblatt International. 2020;**117**(45):764-774. DOI: 10.3238/arztebl.2020.0764

[2] Addiss DG, Shaffer N, Fowler BS, Tauxe RV. The epidemiology of appendicitis and appendectomy in the United States. American Journal of Epidemiology. 1990;**132**(5):910-925. DOI: 10.1093/oxfordjournals.aje.a115734

[3] Gorter RR, Eker HH, Gorter-Stam MA, Abis GS, Acharya A, Ankersmit M, et al. Diagnosis and management of acute appendicitis. EAES consensus development conference. Surgical Endoscopy. 2015;**30**(11):4668-4690. DOI: 10.1007/s00464-016-5245-7

[4] Andersson RE, Petzold MG. Nonsurgical treatment of appendiceal abscess or phlegmon: A systematic review and meta-analysis. Annals of Surgery. 2007;**246**(5):741-748. DOI: 10.1097/SLA.0b013e31811f3f9f

[5] Song CW, Kang JW, Kim JY. Different clinical features and lower scores in clinical scoring systems for appendicitis in preschool children: Comparison with school age onset. Pediatric Gastroenterology, Hepatology & Nutrition. 2018;**21**(1):51-58. DOI: 10.5223/pghn.2018.21.1.51

[6] Gu Nes ME, Deniz MM, Yılmaz S. Diagnostic value of platelet indices in acute appendicitis and comparison with histopathology. Annali Italiani di Chirurgia. 2017;**88**:222-228

[7] Budak YU, Polat M, Huysal K. The use of platelet indices, plateletcrit, mean platelet volume and platelet distribution width in emergency non-traumatic abdominal surgery: A systematic review. Biochemical Medicine (Zagreb). 2016;**26**(2):178-193. DOI: 10.11613/BM.2016.020

[8] Alvarado A. A practical score for the early diagnosis of acute appendicitis. Annals of Emergency Medicine. 1986;**15**(5):557-564. DOI: 10.1016/s0196-0644(86)80993-3

[9] Andersson M, Andersson RE. The appendicitis inflammatory response score: A tool for the diagnosis of acute appendicitis that outperforms the Alvarado score. World Journal of Surgery. 2008;**32**(8):1843-1849. DOI: 10.1007/s00268-008-9649-y

[10] Alotaibi AM, Moshref LH, Moshref RH, Felemban LS. Analysis of 190 female patients after appendectomy. Obstetrics and Gynecology International. 2021;**2021**:8036970. DOI: 10.1155/2021/8036970

[11] Eurboonyanun K, Rungwiriyawanich P, Chamadol N, Promsorn J, Eurboonyanun C, Srimunta P. Accuracy of nonenhanced CT vs contrast-enhanced CT for diagnosis of acute appendicitis in adults. Current Problems in Diagnostic Radiology. 2021;**50**(3):315-320. DOI: 10.1067/j.cpradiol.2020.01.010

[12] Bom WJ, Bolmers MD, Gans SL, van Rossem CC, van Geloven AAW, Bossuyt PMM, et al. Discriminating complicated from uncomplicated appendicitis by ultrasound imaging, computed tomography or magnetic resonance imaging: Systematic review and meta-analysis of diagnostic accuracy. BJS Open. 2021;**5**(2):zraa030. DOI: 10.1093/bjsopen/zraa030

[13] Gaskill CE, Simianu VV, Carnell J, Hippe DS, Bhargava P, Flum DR, et al. Use of computed tomography to determine perforation in patients with acute appendicitis. Current Problems in Diagnostic Radiology. 2018;**47**(1):6-9. DOI: 10.1067/j.cpradiol.2016.12.002

[14] Kim HY, Park JH, Lee YJ, Lee SS, Jeon JJ, Lee KH. Systematic review and meta-analysis of CT features for differentiating complicated and uncomplicated appendicitis. Radiology. 2018;**287**(1):104-115. DOI: 10.1148/radiol.2017171260

[15] Xu Y, Jeffrey RB, Chang ST, DiMaio MA, Olcott EW. Sonographic differentiation of complicated from uncomplicated appendicitis: Implications for antibiotics-first therapy. Journal of Ultrasound in Medicine. 2017;**36**(2):269-277. DOI: 10.7863/ultra.16.03109

[16] Zhang G, Wu B. Meta-analysis of the clinical efficacy of laparoscopic appendectomy in the treatment of acute appendicitis. World Journal of Emergency Surgery: WJES. 2022;**17**(1):26. DOI: 10.1186/s13017-022-00431-1

[17] Masoomi H, Nguyen NT, Dolich MO, Mills S, Carmichael JC, Stamos MJ. Laparoscopic appendectomy trends and outcomes in the United States: Data from the Nationwide Inpatient Sample (NIS), 2004-2011. The American Surgeon. 2014;**80**(10):1074-1077

[18] Liu Y, Cui Z, Zhang R. Laparoscopic versus open appendectomy for acute appendicitis in children. Indian Pediatrics. 2017;**54**(11):938-941. DOI: 10.1007/s13312-017-1186-z

[19] Quah GS, Eslick GD, Cox MR. Laparoscopic appendicectomy is superior to open surgery for complicated appendicitis. Surgical Endoscopy. 2019;**33**(7):2072-2082. DOI: 10.1007/s00464-019-06746-6

[20] Imran JB, Madni TD, Minshall CT, Mokdad AA, Subramanian M, Clark AT, et al. Predictors of a histopathologic diagnosis of complicated appendicitis. The Journal of Surgical Research. 2017;**214**:197-202. DOI: 10.1016/j.jss.2017.02.051

[21] Bastiaenen VP, Allema WM, Klaver CEL, van Dieren S, Koens L, Tanis PJ, et al. Routine histopathologic examination of the appendix after appendectomy for presumed appendicitis: Is it really necessary? A systematic review and meta-analysis. Surgery. 2020;**168**(2):305-312. DOI: 10.1016/j.surg.2020.03.032

[22] Bastiaenen VP, Corten BJ, de Savornin Lohman EA, et al. Safety and cost analysis of selective histopathological examination following appendicectomy and cholecystectomy (FANCY study): Protocol and statistical analysis plan of a prospective observational multicentre study. BMJ Open. 2019;**9**:e035912. DOI: 10.1136/bmjopen-2019-035912

[23] Poprom N, Wilasrusmee C, Attia J, McEvoy M, Thakkinstian A, Rattanasiri S. Comparison of postoperative complications between open and laparoscopic appendectomy: An umbrella review of systematic reviews and meta-analyses. Journal of Trauma and Acute Care Surgery. 2020;**89**(4):813-820. DOI: 10.1097/TA.0000000000002878

[24] Gammeri E, Petrinic T, Bond-Smith G, Gordon-Weeks A. Meta-analysis of peritoneal lavage in appendicectomy. BJS Open. 2018;**3**(1):24-30. DOI: 10.1002/bjs5.50118

[25] Köhler F, Reese L, Kastner C, Hendricks A, Müller S, Lock JF, et al.

Surgical site infection following single-port appendectomy: A systematic review of the literature and meta-analysis. Frontier in Surgery. 2022;**9**:919744. DOI: 10.3389/fsurg.2022.919744

[26] Alotaibi AM, Alfawaz M, Felemban L, Moshref L, Moshref R. Complicated appendicitis increases the hospital length of stay. Surgical Open Science. 2022;**9**:64-68. DOI: 10.1016/j.sopen.2022.05.006

[27] Bailey H. The Ochsner-Sherren (delayed) treatment of acute appendicitis: Indications and technique. British Medical Journal. 1930;**1**(3603):140-143. DOI: 10.1136/bmj.1.3603.140

[28] Coldrey E. Treatment of acute appendicitis. British Medical Journal. 1956;**2**(5007):1458-1461. DOI: 10.1136/bmj.2.5007.1458

[29] Lane JS, Schmit PJ, Chandler CF, Bennion RS, Thompson JE Jr. Ileocecectomy is definitive treatment for advanced appendicitis. The American Surgeon. 2001;**67**(12):1117-1122

[30] Yang Z, Sun F, Ai S, Wang J, Guan W, Liu S. Meta-analysis of studies comparing conservative treatment with antibiotics and appendectomy for acute appendicitis in the adult. BMC Surgery. 2019;**19**(1):110. DOI: 10.1186/s12893-019-0578-5

[31] Podda M, Gerardi C, Cillara N, Fearnhead N, Gomes CA, Birindelli A, et al. Antibiotic treatment and appendectomy for uncomplicated acute appendicitis in adults and children: A systematic review and meta-analysis. Annals of Surgery. 2019;**270**(6):1028-1040. DOI: 10.1097/SLA.0000000000003225

[32] Georgiou R, Eaton S, Stanton MP, Pierro A, Hall NJ. Efficacy and safety of nonoperative treatment for acute appendicitis: A meta-analysis. Pediatrics. 2017;**139**(3):e20163003. DOI: 10.1542/peds.2016-3003

[33] Minneci PC, Hade EM, Lawrence AE, Sebastião YV, Saito JM, Mak GZ, et al. Association of nonoperative management using antibiotic therapy vs laparoscopic appendectomy with treatment success and disability days in children with uncomplicated appendicitis. Journal of the American Medical Association. 2020;**324**(6):581-593. DOI: 10.1001/jama.2020.10888

[34] Salminen P, Tuominen R, Paajanen H, Rautio T, Nordström P, Aarnio M, et al. Five-year follow-up of antibiotic therapy for uncomplicated acute appendicitis in the APPAC Randomized Clinical Trial. JAMA. 2018;**320**(12):1259-1265. DOI: 10.1001/jama.2018.13201. Erratum in: JAMA. 2018 Oct 23;320(16):1711

[35] Herrod PJJ, Kwok AT, Lobo DN. Randomized clinical trials comparing antibiotic therapy with appendicectomy for uncomplicated acute appendicitis: Meta-analysis. BJS Open. 2022;**6**(4):zrac100. DOI: 10.1093/bjsopen/zrac100

[36] Korndorffer JR Jr, Fellinger E, Reed W. SAGES guideline for laparoscopic appendectomy. Surgical Endoscopy. 2010;**24**(4):757-761. DOI: 10.1007/s00464-009-0632-y

[37] Talan DA, Saltzman DJ, DeUgarte DA, Moran GJ. Methods of conservative antibiotic treatment of acute uncomplicated appendicitis: A systematic review. Journal of Trauma and Acute Care Surgery. 2019;**86**(4):722-736. DOI: 10.1097/TA.0000000000002137

[38] Solomkin JS, Mazuski JE, Bradley JS, Rodvold KA, Goldstein EJ, Baron EJ,

et al. Diagnosis and management of complicated intra-abdominal infection in adults and children: Guidelines by the Surgical Infection Society and the Infectious Diseases Society of America. Clinical Infectious Diseases. 2010;**50**(2):133-164. DOI: 10.1086/649554 Erratum in: Clin Infect Dis. 2010 Jun 15;50(12):1695. Dosage error in article text

[39] Mazuski JE, Tessier JM, May AK, Sawyer RG, Nadler EP, Rosengart MR, et al. The surgical infection society revised guidelines on the management of intra-abdominal infection. Surgical Infections. 2017;**18**(1):1-76. DOI: 10.1089/sur.2016.261

[40] Turnbull IR, Horn CB, Guerra J, Punch LJ, Mazuski JE, Bochicchio GV. Twenty-five percent of patients with appendicitis and periappendiceal abscess fail percutaneous drainage alone and require an operation during the Index Hospital Stay. Journal of the American College of Surgeons. 2017;**4**:e80 10.1016/j.jamcollsurg.2017.07.738

[41] Fagenholz PJ, Peev MP, Thabet A, Michailidou M, Chang Y, Mueller PR, et al. Abscess due to perforated appendicitis: Factors associated with successful percutaneous drainage. American Journal of Surgery. 2016;**212**(4):794-798. DOI: 10.1016/j.amjsurg.2015.07.017

[42] Kobayashi S, Makizumi R, Nakahara K, Tsukikawa S, Miyajima N, Otsubo T. Appendiceal abscesses reduced in size by drainage of pus from the appendiceal orifice during colonoscopy: A Report of Three Cases. Case Reports in Gastroenterology. 2014;**8**(3):364-370. DOI: 10.1159/000369549

[43] Ding W, Du Z, Zhou X. Endoscopic retrograde appendicitis therapy for management of acute appendicitis. Surgical Endoscopy. 2022;**36**(4):2480-2487. DOI: 10.1007/s00464-021-08533-8

[44] BouHaidar DS, Bawany MZ, Schubert ML. ERAT: A new era for appendicitis therapy? Digestive Diseases and Sciences. 2016;**61**(11):3099-3101. DOI: 10.1007/s10620-016-4299-7

[45] Gundogar O, Kımıloglu E, Komut N, et al. Evaluation of appendiceal mucinous neoplasms with a new classification system and literature review. The Turkish Journal of Gastroenterology. 2018;**29**:533-542. DOI: 10.5152/tjg.2018.17605

[46] Nagtegaal ID, Odze RD, Klimstra D, Paradis V, Rugge M, Schirmacher P, et al. The 2019 WHO classification of tumours of the digestive system. Histopathology. 2020;**76**(2):182-188. DOI: 10.1111/his.13975

[47] Glasgow SC, Gaertner W, Stewart D, Davids J, Alavi K, Paquette IM, et al. The American Society of Colon and Rectal Surgeons, Clinical Practice Guidelines for the Management of Appendiceal Neoplasms. Diseases of the Colon and Rectum. 2019;**62**(12):1425-1438. DOI: 10.1097/DCR.0000000000001530

[48] Sandor A, Modlin IM. A retrospective analysis of 1570 appendiceal carcinoids. The American Journal of Gastroenterology. 1998;**93**:422-428

[49] Pape UF, Niederle B, Costa F, Gross D, Kelestimur F, Kianmanesh R, et al. ENETS Consensus Guidelines for Neuroendocrine Neoplasms of the Appendix (Excluding Goblet Cell Carcinomas). Neuroendocrinology. 2016;**103**(2):144-152. DOI: 10.1159/000443165

[50] Boudreaux JP, Klimstra DS, Hassan MM, Woltering EA, Jensen RT, Goldsmith SJ, et al. Yao JC;

North American Neuroendocrine Tumor Society (NANETS). The NANETS consensus guideline for the diagnosis and management of neuroendocrine tumors: Well-differentiated neuroendocrine tumors of the Jejunum, Ileum, Appendix, and Cecum. Pancreas. 2010;**39**(6):753-766. DOI: 10.1097/MPA.0b013e3181ebb2a5

[51] Boudreaux JP, Klimstra DS, Hassan MM, Woltering EA, Jensen RT, Goldsmith SJ, et al. The NANETS consensus guideline for the diagnosis and management of neuroendocrine tumors: Well-differentiated neuroendocrine tumors of the Jejunum, Ileum, Appendix, and Cecum. Pancreas. 2010;**39**:753-766

[52] Ricci C, Ingaldi C, Alberici L, Brighi N, Santini D, Mosconi C, et al. Histopathological diagnosis of appendiceal neuroendocrine neoplasms: When to perform a right hemicolectomy? A systematic review and meta-analysis. Endocrine. 2019;**66**(3):460-466. DOI: 10.1007/s12020-019-01984-z

[53] Nonaka D, Papaxoinis G, Lamarca A, Fulford P, Valle J, Chakrabarty B. A study of appendiceal crypt cell adenocarcinoma (so-called goblet cell carcinoid and its related adenocarcinoma). Human Pathology. 2018;**72**:18-27. DOI: 10.1016/j.humpath.2017.08.005

[54] Palmer K, Weerasuriya S, Chandrakumaran K, Rous B, White BE, Paisey S, et al. Goblet cell adenocarcinoma of the Appendix: A systematic review and incidence and survival of 1,225 cases from an English Cancer Registry. Frontiers in Oncology. 2022;**12**:915028. DOI: 10.3389/fonc.2022.915028

Chapter 10

Nursing Management of Patients with Appendicitis

Vivian E.A. Eta, Nahyeni Bassah, Malika Esembeson and John Ngunde Palle

Abstract

Acute appendicitis is a common emergency in general surgery and globally appendectomy is at the top of emergency surgical procedures. Evidence suggests appendectomy is the first-line treatment for acute appendicitis. About 9% of patients develop complications after appendectomy, leading to a long hospital stay and recurrent surgery among others. Surgical site infection (SSI) is a common complication of appendectomy. Many factors may contribute to the occurrence of SSI either during preoperative, intraoperative, or postoperative periods. The important role nurses play in the management of appendicitis from admission to discharge cannot be underestimated. This chapter describes nursing assessment, diagnoses and the care plan for a patient with appendicitis on admission. Also, the role of the nurse play during preoperative, intraoperative and postoperative periods, and at Discharge are presented. This information could improve the quality of care and reduce complications.

Keywords: appendicitis, appendectomy, preoperative, postoperative, nursing assessment, nursing diagnoses, nursing care plan

1. Introduction

The vermiform appendix is a thin, tube-like organ attached to the cecum and has lymphatic tissues that control infection. Appendicitis, also called epityphlitis, is the inflammation of the appendix, a small finger-like appendage attached to the cecum found just below the ileocecal valve. In other words, appendicitis is an acute inflammation of the vermiform appendix. Acute appendicitis is the most common abdominal surgical emergency, with an incidence of almost 100 per 100,000 people in Australia, Europe, and North America [1]. Appendicitis is common among the age group between 10 and 30 years [2].

An individual with appendicitis complains of vague epigastric or periumbilical pain, which progresses to the right lower quadrant generally accompanied by low-grade fever, anorexia, nausea, and sometimes vomiting. In 50% of patients, local tenderness is elicited at McBurney's point, when pressure is applied [3]. Also, there is rebound tenderness or the production or intensification of pain when pressure is released. In addition, Rovsing's sign may be elicited by palpating the left lower quadrant; this unexpectedly causes pain to be felt in the right lower quadrant.

Furthermore, there is elevated white blood cell count, client taking the side-lying position, as well as constipation or diarrhea. These symptoms may indicate uncomplicated appendicitis.

For complicated appendicitis the patient experiences severe abdominal pain, which prevents movement, the patient holds his/her abdomen very still and avoids deep breaths. Also, the abdomen feels very firm to touch due to abdominal guarding, legs are flexed, and the patient presents with fever (37.7°C [100° F] or greater) and toxic appearance. These symptoms could indicate a ruptured appendix, which might result in peritonitis or appendicular abscess. Some of the predisposing factors are obstruction by fecalith or foreign bodies, bacteria or toxins, low-fiber diet, and high intake of refined carbohydrates [4].

Usually, diagnosis of appendicitis is based on a comprehensive physical examination, laboratory and radiologic tests, and the treatment is by appendectomy. Appendectomy is the surgical removal of the vermiform appendix and evidence suggests it is the first-line treatment for acute appendicitis globally [5]. Nonetheless, antibiotic therapy may be effective for a selected group of patients with uncomplicated acute appendicitis. It is important to state that appendectomy is a relatively safe surgical intervention with a case fatality rate of 2.1–2.4 per 1000 patients, as reported in studies conducted in Europe [2, 3, 6]. However, about 9% of patients develop complications after appendectomy leading to a long hospital stay and recurrent surgery among others. Surgical site infection (SSI) is a common complication of appendectomy [7]. Many factors may contribute to the occurrence of SSI either during preoperative, intraoperative, or postoperative periods. The important role nurses play in the management of appendicitis from admission to discharge cannot be underestimated.

This chapter describes nursing assessment, diagnoses, and the care plan for a patient with appendicitis on admission. Also, the role of the nurse play during preoperative, intraoperative and postoperative periods, and at discharge are presented. This information could improve the quality of care and reduce complications among patients.

2. Nursing assessment, nursing diagnoses, and the care plan on admission

Adequate nursing assessment and diagnoses are necessary on admission for proper planning and implementing a patient-centered quality nursing care. The following subsection presents guidelines for conducting nursing assessments and formulating diagnoses for patients with appendicitis.

2.1 Nursing assessment and diagnoses

On admission, the nurse is expected to assess the patient presenting with the signs and symptoms of appendicitis in order to formulate nursing diagnoses, plan, and implement quality care. A comprehensive and systematic health assessment that is completed within a reasonable time frame remains one of the most significant components of patient care and cannot be underestimated [8]. The comprehensive health assessment (also known as complete or initial health assessment) is made up of a thorough health history taking (interview with the patient) and physical examination, which is often done when the patient is stable. The initial health assessment is conducted to obtain the patient's baseline information, which is very vital in monitoring the patient and evaluating interventions implemented [9].

This is done by questioning the patient about chief complaint, and past and current symptoms as well as reviewing the patient's past medical and surgical records, including family history and lifestyle. A thorough physical examination is then conducted to determine if the Rovsing's sign is positive [10]. The nurse palpates the left lower quadrant of the abdomen and asks the patient if this action increases the pain felt in the right lower quadrant. Also, (s)he applies pressure at McBurney's point to ascertain if it is tender and then checks for rebound tenderness (if the pain is intensified when pressure is released) [11].

The severity of the pain is then determined and the patient's vital signs are checked and recorded. Furthermore, relevant laboratory findings are reviewed (results may reveal an elevated white blood cell count of above 10,000 per cubic millimeter, while abdominal radiographs, ultrasound studies, and CT scans may reveal right lower quadrant density or localized distention of the bowel) [12]. It is important to note that the comprehensive health assessment may indicate a problem-focused assessment, which is often done when a potential health problem has been identified [13].

The information gathered from the complete health assessment is then synthesized, analyzed, and documented. Another type of assessment that may still be performed is the interval (abbreviated) health assessment, which should be conducted after obtaining baseline data from the comprehensive assessment [14]. The nurse usually performs an interval (abbreviated) assessment at change of shift, when the patient returns from tests, or upon transfer to another unit (i.e., from the theater to the surgical unit) as well as at subsequent visits on an outpatient basis (see Section 4.3.1).

It is worth stating that for the health assessment to be thorough, the nurse is expected to communicate appropriately with the patient and performs a culturally sensitive physical examination [15]. This helps to elicit the required information needed for proper planning and the provision of quality nursing care. The subsequent section presents some guidelines for conducting a thorough health assessment for all patients with appendicitis including those with disabilities.

2.1.1 Guidelines for performing nursing assessment and formulating diagnoses

The health assessment of a patient with appendicitis may gather both objective and subjective; hence, good interviewing and physical examination skills are mandatory. Thus, the following subsections provide guidelines for conducting health assessments and stating nursing diagnoses.

2.1.1.1 Principles guiding the conduct of health assessments

When conducting health assessments, the nurse should:

- Be prepared to accommodate special needs persons and conduct a culturally sensitive assessment.

- Take into consideration the psychosocial, physical, emotional, environmental, cultural, and spiritual factors that might influence the procedure.

- Adapt the environment (examination room, table, etc.) accordingly to suit those with various disabilities; minimize noise, colors, smells, and bright lights as needed.
- Get all necessary equipment handy to avoid wasting time and causing exhaustion.
- Modify the physical exam techniques employed for the procedure accordingly for each individual, especially those with disabilities.
- Demonstrate effective communication (verbal and nonverbal) and interviewing skills, which establish an atmosphere of trust and respect at the beginning and throughout the procedure. Adapt different modes of communication where necessary, keeping speech slow and alternating tone as required.
- Introduce yourself and obtain consent from the patient before proceeding with the assessment.
- Appropriately and adequately assist patients needing help with completing hospital forms, undressing, climbing, and going down from examination tables.
- Avoid being judgmental and show respect for each patient's culture.
- Be patient and treat patient with courtesy, avoid harm or repeating harmful maneuvers.
- Observe proper hygiene practices to control infection, ensures patient's privacy, and use draping as required as well as maintain confidentiality.
- Employ the recommended framework for history taking and physical examination while making modifications to accommodate patients with disabilities.
- Exhibit skills to appropriately distinguish between normal, variations of normal, and abnormal findings in patient data recognizing while influential factors and their clinical significance.
- Demonstrate skills in documenting and describing verbally the findings of the health assessment in a format appropriate for proper and accurate communication in the multidisciplinary health care setting.

2.1.1.2 Guidelines for formulating and stating nursing diagnoses

Clinical decision-making and diagnostic reasoning are approaches to support the identification of a patient's problem. The nurse applies his/her clinical decision-making skills to synthesize health assessment information, use critical inquiry and clinical reasoning to diagnose health risks, and differentiate signs of health from ill health [16]. The information gathered is compared to norms and standards, organized according to a predetermined structure, and subsequently interpreted yielding individualized strengths and limitations from which a problem list is created.

Identifying the problem enables the nurse to initiate the treatment plan [17]. Thus, after listing the problems, appropriate interventions are planned, implemented and continually evaluated, and revised to assist the patient to achieve and maintain optimal health.

2.2 The nursing care plan for the patient with appendicitis on admission

Usually, the nurse is expected to prioritize the patient's problems and draw up a nursing care plan to focus on life-threatening symptoms. In drawing up the care plan, the following components are taken into account; the nursing diagnoses, goals to be achieved, interventions, the expected outcomes, and evaluation to determine if the interventions were effective [18]. Below are presented these different aspects.

2.2.1 Nursing diagnoses

Generally, based on the assessment data, the most appropriate diagnoses for a patient with appendicitis on admission and before appendectomy would probably be [19]:

- Pain (acute) related to obstructed appendix /inflammation due to distension of intestinal tissues as evidenced by expressive behavior (e.g., restlessness, moaning, crying, vigilance, irritability, and sighing).

- Risk for deficient fluid volume related to preoperative vomiting evidenced by poor skin turgor.

- Risk for infection related to a ruptured appendix, peritonitis, and abscess formationevidenced by the disruption of the GI tract.

- Risk for malnutrition related to anorexia and nausea evidenced by less-than-body requirements.

2.2.2 Planning interventions

This stage starts with stating the goals to be achieved for a patient with appendicitis, based on the problems identified [20], these include; to:

- Relieve pain.

- Prevent fluid volume deficit.

- Reduce anxiety.

- Eliminate infection due to the potential or actual disruption of the GI tract.

- Maintain skin integrity.

- Attain optimal nutrition.

The plan for care should be negotiated with patients and their caregivers to ensure clear expectations and compliance with the nursing interventions [21].

2.2.3 Implementing nursing interventions

2.2.3.1 Uncomplicated appendicitis

Based on the stated goals of the nurse:

- Administers analgesics (Opioids) as prescribed respecting the route and frequency of administration.
- Administers fluids as prescribed to replace fluid loss and promote adequate renal functioning while monitoring the patient for fluid overload. Oral fluids when tolerated, could be administered.
- Administers antibiotics (e.g., ceftriaxone) as prescribed.
- Educates the patient about his/her condition to reduce anxiety.
- Ensures daily baths (body hygiene).
- Serves well-balanced meals.
- Monitors patient closely for signs of improvement.
- Immediately reports abnormal findings.

2.2.3.2 Complicated appendicitis

For complicated cases, in addition to the above interventions the nurse:

- Administers the required analgesics strictly respecting the route and frequency of administration as well as uses non-pharmacological measures to reduce severe pain or discomfort (see Section 3.1 for details).
- Monitors the patient closely for signs of perforation and peritonitis such as if the abdomen appears to be very firm and tender to touch.
- Should alert the physician immediately if signs of perforation and peritonitis are evident.
- Should closely monitor vital signs to determine sudden changes, such as increased heart rate (tachycardia) or fever, as this could indicate infection or acute inflammation.
- Should check and empty drain if put in place preoperatively, and provide appropriate and adequate care.
- Reports signs of infection.
- Prepares the patient for surgery as required.

2.2.4 Expected or desired outcomes

After implementing the intervention, the nurse:

- Expects the patient to report a reduction in pain.
- Documents adequate hydration.
- Reports no signs of infection.
- Documents reduced level of anxiety.
- Reports intact skin.
- Documents adequate nutrition.

2.2.5 Evaluation

The outcomes of the interventions are evaluated to ensure the goals are achieved as expected [22]. For instance:

- The patient verbalized reduction in pain.
- The nurse documented normal fluid volume.
- The nurse noticed reduced level of anxiety.
- The nurse reported no signs of infection.
- The nurse reported intact skin.
- The nurse recorded adequate nutrition.

In addition, the nurse continues to monitor the patient and be alert to identify, intervene or report any new symptom(s) that may come up. Hence, other nursing responsibilities include vital signs monitoring, assisting the patient to do laboratory investigations as required, reviewing laboratory findings, and acting accordingly [23]. Above all, the nurse is expected to prepare the patient for surgery (see Section 5.1). Since abnormal laboratory findings are indications of illness progression, the nurse should:

a. Review laboratory results to identify abnormal values, such as:

  - CRP >1 mg/dL, which indicates inflammation, very high levels may indicate gangrene.
  - WBC >10,500, which indicates infection.

b. The nurse should closely monitor the patient with the following in mind:

- That fever, chills, and diaphoresis are signs of infection, eminent sepsis, abscess, or peritonitis.

- Hypotension with tachycardia may indicate dehydration if vomiting or diarrhea is severe.

It is important to note that pain, which is the main symptom of appendicitis, can be controlled by the use of pharmacological as well as non-pharmacological measures [24]. The next section presents these details.

2.3 Relieving pain through non-pharmacologic interventions

There are a variety of nursing actions that are undertaken to relieve a patient's pain. These include distraction techniques, positioning, and application of ice bags among others [25]. The non-pharmacological methods for relieving pain in a patient with appendicitis are presented below.

1. Placing the patient in a semi-Fowler's position: After the surgery, the nurse places the patient in a High-fowler's position to reduce the tension on the incision and abdominal organs, thereby reducing pain. This position allows gravity to assist by reducing abdominal stress and relieving discomfort [4].

2. Applying ice bag on the abdomen periodically during the first 24- to 48-hour period as required. This intervention soothes and relieves pain through the desensitization of nerve endings [26].

3. Educating and assisting the patient to protect the abdomen before and after surgery by splinting with a pillow while coughing or engaging in any stressful activity. This will aid in pain reduction and prevent the dehiscence of an incision.

2.4 Dos and do nots during nursing interventions

It is worth mentioning that there are some nursing interventions that must not be performed on the patient with appendicitis because of their harmful consequences [27]. The dos and do nots at admission, pre- and postoperative periods regarding a patient with appendicitis are stated below.

2.4.1 Dos

The nurse should:

- Administer analgesics judiciously before the diagnosis of appendicitis. This may mask the symptom of pain.

- Administer regular analgesia after appendicitis has been diagnosed, usually, an opioid depending on pain severity is given to make the patient comfortable before health assessment.

- Recommend the use of mild laxatives or stool softeners as necessary. This may assist with a return to usual bowel function and prevents undue straining for defecation.

- Monitor the patient closely to identify signs of rupture.
- Give the patient nothing by mouth several hours before surgery.
- Place the ice bag on the abdomen periodically during the first 24- to 48-hour period as required. This intervention soothes and relieves pain through the desensitization of nerve endings.
- Maintain NPO status after surgery until bowel function has returned.
- Advance diet gradually as tolerated or as prescribed when bowel sounds return.

2.4.2 Do nots

The nurse should not:

- Apply any heat over the area of pain while the patient is awaiting diagnosis as this could cause the appendix to rupture.
- Use heat on the patient's right lower abdomen, because it may cause tissue congestion.
- Administer enemas as they may induce peristalsis, which may cause perforation.
- Administer analgesia before examination because this can lead to an inaccurate diagnosis as the pain may subside and the examination will be ineffective.

3. Nursing assessment and interventions during preoperative and postoperative periods

These periods are crucial for the patient and the health care team as it determines the patient's outcome [28]. The specific nursing activities during the preoperative and postoperative periods are discussed in the subsequent sections.

3.1 Nursing interventions during preoperative period

The nurse needs to prepare the patient several hours presurgery. Generally, during this period the main goal is to prepare the patient adequately for surgery (appendectomy) in order to ensure a successful surgery and a positive outcome post-surgery [29]. However, the abbreviated health assessment may be conducted on the patient if needed. This will help to identify symptoms that were not present at admission and those missed during routine care after admission so that necessary actions could be taken accordingly. For instance, the patient may be dehydrated due to continuous nausea and vomiting [30], and or might be anxious probably due to inadequate information regarding condition and surgery. Thus, the nurse is expected to intervene accordingly while observing the patient closely. Depending on local policies, the nurse:

- Maintains patent IV hydration to continuously replace fluid loss as needed, and promote adequate renal functioning.

- Thoroughly explains the procedure to the patient and obtain informed consent.
- Educates the patient on pre- and postoperative care/activities.
- Cleans and shaves the operation site before surgery.
- Initiates NPO status to empty gastric contents if indicated.
- Assesses (monitors for changes in the level of pain) and continues to manage pain.
- Places an ice pack on RLQ to aid in pain relief every hour for 20–30 minutes as prescribed.
- Encourages abdominal splinting to control pain.
- Encourages bed rest.
- Continues to administer antibiotic prophylaxis to prevent infection.
- Monitors for signs of a ruptured appendix.
- Administers medication if necessary to lower an elevated temperature.
- Assesses relevant laboratory findings.
- Assesses and records the patient's vital signs in preparation for surgery.
- Positions the patient in right-side lying or semi-fowler position to promote comfort.
- Monitors bowel sounds.

3.2 The role of the nurse during surgery

The role nurses play during surgery cannot be overemphasized. The nurse acts as the scrub nurse, instrument nurse, or circulating nurse as well as assisting the surgeon directly during surgery [31]. The scrub nurse also known as the instrument nurse sets up the sterile field observing strict aseptic techniques. She/he assists the surgeon to scrub and dress into his/her theater wear, and hands surgical instruments to the surgeon during surgery. The instrument nurse is a member of the sterile team who scrubs, gowns, and gloves for the surgical procedure. She is responsible for setting up and handing sterile supplies and instruments to the surgeon [32].

The circulating nurse oversees nursing care during the procedure and ensures that the operating room remains sterile. Responsibilities include ensuring that surgical asepsis is adhered to during the surgical procedure, keeping track and conducting an inventory of supplies and equipment used during and after the surgical procedure, or calling for a time-out [33]. An operating nurse also acts as a liaison between the patient, the patient's relatives, and the medical team. In addition, the nurse can also function as an anesthetics, she/he assesses the patient, administers anesthesia, and monitors the patient closely during surgery.

3.3 Postoperative nursing assessment, diagnoses, and interventions

3.3.1 Postoperative nursing assessment

Generally, after surgery, the nurse performs an abbreviated health assessment (and then a focused health assessment if indicated) in order to produce a list of the patient's problems. The abbreviated health assessment is not as detailed as the complete assessment that occurs at admission. The advantage of an abbreviated assessment is that at this time it allows the nurse to thoroughly assess the surgical patient in a shorter period of time [34]. The problem-focused assessment may be conducted if a new symptom emerges, or the patient develops any distress.

The focused health assessment focuses on a specific injury or medical complaint and vital signs, which include pulse, respirations, skin signs, pupils, and blood pressure. In conducting the focused health assessment, the nurse focuses the physical examination on that specific injury or new complaint [35]. Generally, in a focused physical examination, only the requested body part or system is examined. After the assessment, the nursing priorities in the postoperative period mainly include:

1. Prevent complications.

2. Promote comfort.

3. Provide information about surgical procedure/prognosis, treatment needs, and potential complications.

The nurse uses the care plan to achieve all of the above in the postoperative period as shown below.

3.3.2 Postoperative nursing diagnoses and interventions

Note; the procedure for formulating the nursing diagnoses is as stated above (see Section 2.2).

3.3.2.1 Nursing diagnoses, goals, and desired (expected) outcomes

After the health assessment, the nursing diagnoses (ND) should be prioritized as follows:

- ND-1: Acute pain related to surgical incision evidenced by [36]:

  - Complaints of pain.

  - Facial grimacing and muscle guarding.

  - Expressive behavior (restlessness, moaning, and crying).

  - Autonomic responses.

The goal is to reduce pain and increase comfort.

- Desired outcomes; the patient should:
  - Report reduced pain.
  - Appear relaxed, able to sleep, and rest appropriately.
  - Demonstrate the use of relaxation techniques and diversional activities, as indicated for an individual situation.

ND-2: Risk for fluid volume deficit related possibly to [37]:

- Preoperative vomiting and postoperative restrictions (e.g., NPO);
- Hypermetabolic state (e.g., fever, healing process);
- Inflammation of peritoneum with sequestration of fluid evidenced by:

The goal is to maintain adequate fluid intake and output.

- Desired outcomes.
- The nurse should document the following within a reasoning time frame [38]:
  - Adequate hydration (by IV fluids)/fluid balance as evidenced by moist mucous membranes, good skin turgor, stable vital signs, and normal urine input & output chart.

ND-3: Risk for infection related to surgery and surgical site, and inadequate primary defenses evidenced by fever, inflammation, and pus at the surgical site [39].

The goal is to prevent infection.

- Desired outcomes; the nurse should document:
  - Timely wound healing with no signs of infection/inflammation, purulent drainage, erythema, and fever.
- ND-4: Deficient knowledge probably related to:
  - Inability to recall information or information misinterpretation.
  - Unfamiliarity with information resources.

All evidenced possibly by:

- Questions; request for information; and verbalization of problem/concerns.
- Statement of misconception.
- Inaccurate follow-through of instruction.

- Development of preventable complications.

The goal is to provide adequate information on the condition and reduce anxiety. Desired outcomes, the patient should:

- Verbalize understanding of disease process and potential complications.
- Verbalize understanding of therapeutic needs.
- Participate in the treatment regimen.

3.3.2.2 Nursing interventions

The nursing interventions (NI) for the stated problems are presented below accordingly NI-1; the nurse should do the following:

Assess pain, noting location, characteristics, and severity (on a scale of 0–10), then investigate and report changes in pain as appropriate. This is important in determining the effectiveness of medication and the progression of healing [40]. The nurse should:

- Provide accurate, honest information to patients and families, this helps to decrease anxiety.
- Use non-pharmacological measures to reduce pain.
- Encourage early ambulation, this helps to normalize organ function (stimulates peristalsis and passing of flatus, reducing abdominal discomfort). For an immobile patient, serial compression devices (SCD) and TED hose should be used to avoid DVT clots.
- Provide diversional activities; this refocuses the patient's attention, promotes relaxation, and may enhance coping abilities.
- Keep NPO and maintain NG suction initially(if inserted), this minimizes the discomfort of early intestinal peristalsis, gastric irritation, and vomiting.
- Administer analgesics as prescribed, this helps to relieve pain and enhances cooperation with other therapeutic interventions (such as ambulation and pulmonary toilet).
- Place the ice bag on the abdomen during the first 24–48-hour period as required. This intervention soothes and relieves pain through the desensitization of nerve endings.
- Watch closely for possible signs of surgical complications; continuous pain, inflammation, and fever may signal surgical site infection

NI-2; the nurse should do the following:

- Monitor BP and pulse; changes in these parameters help identify fluctuating intravascular volumes.

- Inspect mucous membranes, and assess skin turgor and capillary refill; these indicate if peripheral circulation and cellular hydration are adequate.

- Monitor input and output noting the color of urine and concentration, as well as specific gravity. It is worth stating that decreasing output of concentrated urine with increasing specific gravity indicates dehydration and the need for increased fluids [41].

- Auscultate and document bowel sounds noting the passing of flatus and bowel movement. These are pointers of the return of peristalsis, and readiness to begin oral intake. Note for a patient who has had a laparoscopic procedure and been discharged in less than 24 hours, this may not happen in the hospital [42].

- Provide clear liquids in small amounts when oral intake is indicated, and progress to liquid, then semi-liquid diet and solids as tolerated. This reduces the risk of gastric irritation and vomiting, which minimizes fluid loss.

- Give frequent mouth care with special attention to the protection of the lips. This is because dehydration results in drying and painful cracking of the lips and mouth [43].

- Continue administering IV fluids and electrolytes as needed. This is because the peritoneum reacts to irritation and infection by producing large amounts of intestinal fluid, possibly reducing the circulating blood volume, resulting in dehydration and relative electrolyte imbalances.

NI-3; the nurse should do the following:

- Administer antibiotics (e.g., ceftriaxone and metronidazole IV as prescribed.

- Dress the incision side using a strict aseptic technique.

- Monitor temperature for signs of infection.

- Assess the incision for signs of infection, such as redness, swelling, and pain.

NI-4; the nurse should:

- Identify symptoms requiring medical evaluation (e.g., increasing pain; edema or erythema of wound; the presence of drainage, fever). The timely intervention will reduce the risk of serious complications, such as delayed wound healing and peritonitis [44].

- Review postoperative activity restrictions that are, heavy lifting, exercise, sex, sports, and driving. This is in order to assist the patient to plan for a return to usual routines without untoward incidents.

- Encourage the patient to return to normal activities progressively as tolerated with periodic rest periods. This will prevent fatigue, promote healing and feeling of well-being, and enable the patient to return to normal activities without complications.

- Discuss care of the incision, including dressing changes, bathing restrictions, and removing sutures as indicated. This will enhance compliance with the therapeutic regimen, and promotes the healing and recovery process [45].

- Encourage the patient to cough, breathe deeply, and turn frequently in order to prevent pulmonary complication

Other important nursing responsibilities during the postoperative period

- The nurse ensures that during the postoperative period vital signs are regularly monitored that is, every 30 minutes for 2 hours, and every hour for 2 hours. If the patient is stable, vital signs monitoring should be done every 4 hours while the patient is recovering in the hospital.

- The nurse makes sure for patients who have had a straightforward appendectomy the surgical team should review them on recovery and decides when they may eat and drink.

- The nurse is expected to record input and output daily as well as the output of the drain if the drain was inserted during surgery. Consider removing the drain when minimal drainage is noticed; usually 50 ml or less.

- The nurse uses aseptic techniques to care for the wound; if the wound is covered with a dry dressing, it should be changed every 1–2 days [46]. The clips or stitches should be removed after 10 days of surgery except if indicated otherwise. The patient may be discharged home with stitches in place; hence, the patient might be told to return for removal or referred to the nearest health facility. If dissolvable stitches were used, the patient is told when to come back for the wound to be accessed.

- The nurse encourages the patient to get up and out of bed as soon as possible (*ambulation*) to prevent the formation of emboli. Anticoagulants are usually administered in the form of subcutaneous injections before surgery and postoperatively.

- The nurse encourages the patient to wear anti-embolism stockings and *deep breathing and coughing exercises.*

- The nurse should be aware of the following:

- The convalescence period is almost invariably smooth and the patient recovers rapidly.

- The hospital stay for patients who have undergone an uncomplicated appendectomy is usually 2–3 days.

- In most cases, the patient will be discharged when their temperature is normal and their bowels have started to function again.

- The nurse educates the patient and significant others during this period on how to continue care at home, for instance, proper wound care, nutrition (*proper high fiber, protein, and vitamin C diets*), hygiene, and exercise among others.

4. Discharge procedure and the role of the nurse

The nurse has the duty to ensure that before discharge, the patient is confident in how to continue care for the incision site at home and has details of who to contact in case of any concern [47]. Generally, before discharge, the patient is assessed and the incision site checked for signs of healing and the outcome will determine whether the patient is to be discharged or not.

4.1 Patient and family teaching on home care and prevention of complications

Discharge teaching for patient and family is mandatory; therefore, the nurse is expected to educate the patient on the following before discharge:

- When the sutures will be removed: The nurse discusses with the patient to return for the removal of the sutures (if still in place).

- Medications to be taken at home if any: The nurse explains to the patient how each medication is to be taken, dosage, frequency, and duration, and side effects to watch for and report as necessary.

- How to return to normal activities: Heavy lifting is to be avoided postoperatively; however, normal activity can be resumed gradually within 2 to 4 weeks.

- Proper hygiene practices: The nurse educates on good hand washing and perineal care.

- Wound care: A home care nurse may be needed to assist with the care of the surgical site if available, and to monitor the patient for complications and wound healing (or signs of infection). If not the patient and family are educated on aseptic wound care to prevent infection.

- Nutrition: Instruct the patient that diet can be advanced to her or his normal food pattern as long as no gastrointestinal distress is experienced. What class of food and proportion to take frequently to enhance healing and maintain good health is mentioned.

- Preventing/minimizing complications: The nurse informs the patient that a possible complication of appendicitis is peritonitis, and discusses with the patient symptoms that indicate peritonitis, such as sharp abdominal pains, fever, nausea and vomiting, and increased pulse and respiration. The patient must seek medical attention immediately should these symptoms occur.

- Meeting needs after discharge: The nurse plans with the patient on how to report new complaints.

5. Conclusion

Appendicitis is an acute inflammation of the vermiform appendix, which is the cause of the most common abdominal surgical emergency with minimal complications. However, surgical action should be taken without delay. If left untreated there is a risk of peritonitis, which is the main complication of this condition. Some signs and symptoms of appendicitis are a pain in the right lower quadrant of the abdomen. Nurses play a significant role in the management of appendicitis from admission to discharge. Understanding the nurse's responsibilities at admission, pre- and post-surgery is very vital for proper nursing interventions and good outcomes. Nurses are expected to use good clinical decision and clinical reasoning skills to analyze and synthesize patient data in order to prioritize patient problems, set goals, and plan and implement patient-centered care.

Author details

Vivian E.A. Eta[1*], Nahyeni Bassah[1], Malika Esembeson[1,2] and John Ngunde Palle[1]

1 Faculty of Health Sciences, Department of Nursing, University of Buea, Buea, Cameroon

2 Faculty of Health Sciences, Department of Public Health and Hygiene, University of Buea, Buea, Cameroon

*Address all correspondence to: ayambaenow@yahoo.com

References

[1] Poillucci G, Mortola L, Podda M, Di Saverio S, Casula L, Gerardi C, et al. Laparoscopic appendectomy vs antibiotic therapy for acute appendicitis: A propensity score-matched analysis from a multicenter cohort study. Updates in Surgery. 2017;**69**(4):531-540. DOI: 10.1007/s13304-017-0499-8

[2] Feng J, Cui N, Wang Z, Duan J. Bayesian network meta-analysis of the effects of single-incision laparoscopic surgery, conventional laparoscopic appendectomy and open appendectomy for the treatment of acute appendicitis. Experimental and Therapeutic Medicine. 2017;**14**(6):5908-5916. DOI: 10.3892/etm.2017.5343

[3] Leary DP, Walsh SM, Bolger J, Baban C, Humphreys H, Grady S, et al. A randomized clinical trial evaluating the efficacy and quality of life of antibiotic-only treatment of acute uncomplicated appendicitis: Results of the COMMA trial. Annals of Surgery. 2021;**274**(2):240-247. DOI: 10.1097/SLA.0000000000004785

[4] Bhangu A, Søreide K, Di Saverio S, Assarsson JH, Drake FT. Acute appendicitis: Modern understanding of pathogenesis, diagnosis, and management. Lancet. 2015;**386**(10000):1278-1287. DOI: 10.1016/S0140-6736(15)00275-5

[5] Di Saverio S, Podda M, De Simone B, Ceresoli M, Augustin G, Gori A, et al. Diagnosis and treatment of acute appendicitis: 2020 update of the WSES Jerusalem guidelines. World Journal of Emergency Surgery : WJES. 2020;**15**(1):1-42. DOI: 10.1186/s13017-020-00306-3

[6] Snyder MJ, Guthrie M, Cagle S. Acute appendicitis: Efficient diagnosis and management. American Family Physician. 2018;**98**(1):25-33 PMID: 30215950

[7] Köhler F, Reese L, Kastner C, Hendricks A, Müller S, Lock JF, et al. Surgical site infection following single-port Appendectomy: A systematic review of the literature and Meta-analysis. Frontiers in Surgery. 2022;**9**:919744. DOI: 10.3389/fsurg.2022.919744

[8] Berman A, Snyder S, Kozier B, Erb G. Erb's Fundamentals of Nursing: Concepts, Process, and Practice. 9th ed. Upper Saddle River, N.J: Pearson Education, Inc; 2012

[9] Toney-Butler TJ, Unison-Pace, WJ. Nursing Admission Assessment and Examination. 2022. Available from: https://www.ncbi.nlm.nih.gov/books/NBK493211/ [Accessed: December 1, 2022]

[10] Mock K, Lu Y, Friedlander S, Kim DY, Lee SL. Misdiagnosing adult appendicitis: Clinical, cost, and socioeconomic implications of negative appendectomy. American Journal of Surgery. 2016;**212**(6):1076-1082. DOI: 10.1016/j.amjsurg.2016.09.005

[11] Bhangu A, Søreide K, Di Saverio S, et al. Acute appendicitis: Modern understanding of pathogenesis, diagnosis, and management. Lancet. 2015;**386**:1278-1287

[12] Harnoss JC, Zelienka I, Probst P, Grummich K, Müller-Lantzsch C, Harnoss JM, et al. Antibiotics versus surgical therapy for uncomplicated appendicitis: Systematic review and meta-analysis of controlled trials (PROSPERO 2015:CRD42015016882).

Annals of Surgery. 2017;**265**(5):889-900. DOI: 10.1097/SLA.0000000000002039

[13] Bickley L. Bates' Visual Guide to Physical Examination. 5th ed. Philadelphia, PA: Wolters Kluwer; 2013

[14] Edmunds L, Ward S, Barnes R. The use of advanced physical assessment skills by cardiac nurses. British Journal of Nursing. 2010;**19**(5):282-287

[15] Caple C. Physical Assessment: Performing- Cultural Considerations. Glendale, CA: Cinahl Information Systems; 2011

[16] Susan G, Sonia H, Clint M, Nicholas R. Characteristics and processes of clinical reasoning in nurses and factors related to its use: A scoping review protocol. JBI Database of Systematic Reviews and Implementation Reports. 2017;**15**(12):2832-2836. DOI: 10.11124/JBISRIR-2016-003273

[17] Young ME, Thomas A, Lubarsky S, et al. Mapping clinical reasoning literature across the health professions: A scoping review. BMC Medical Education. 2020;**20**:107. DOI: 10.1186/s12909-020-02012-9

[18] Gaines K. How to conduct a nursing head-to-toe assessment. Available from: https://nurse.org/articles/how-to-conduct-head-to-toe-assessment/ [Accessed: December 1, 2022]

[19] Jones MW, Lopez RA, Deppen JG, Kendall BA 2022. Appendicitis (Nursing). Available from: https://www.ncbi.nlm.nih.gov/books/NBK568712/. [Accessed: December 1, 2022]

[20] Nursing path. Appendicitis Management and Nursing Care Plan 2018. Avilable from: https://www.nursingpath.in/2018/05/appendicitis-management-and-nursing.html [Accessed: December 1, 2022]

[21] Dunham M, MacInnes J. Relationship of multiple attempts on an admissions examination to early program performance. The Journal of Nursing Education. 2018;**57**(10):578-583

[22] Gray LC, Beattie E, Boscart VM, Henderson A, Hornby-Turner YC, Hubbard RE, et al. Development and testing of the interRAI acute care: A standardized assessment administered by nurses for patients admitted to acute care. Health Service Insights. 2018;**11**:1178

[23] Eta Vivian EA, Palle JN, Nsagha DS, Nana NTand Atemnkeng NC. Nurses' knowledge and practices regarding factors associated with surgical site infection and nursing management. African Journal of Integration Health. 2018;**08**(01):28-32

[24] Gillespie B, Chaboyer W, Kang E, Hewitt J, Niuewenhoven P, Morely N. Postsurgery wound assessment and management practices: A chart audit. Journal of Clinical Nursing. 2014;**2014**. DOI: 10.1111/jocn.12574

[25] Harris CL, Kuhnke J, Haley J, Cross K, Somayaji R, Dubois J, et al. Best practice recommendations for the prevention and management of surgical wound complications. Canadian Association of Wound Care. 2018:1-66

[26] Wagner M. Appendicitis Nursing Diagnosis & Care Plan. 2022. Available from: https://www.nursetogether.com/abdominal-pain-nursing-diagnosis-care-plan/ [Accessed: December 2, 2022]

[27] RNspeak. Appendectomy Nursing Care Plan. 2022. Available from: https://rnspeak.com/appendectomy-nursing-care-plan/ [Accessed: December 2, 2022]

[28] Awuviry N. Effects of NPR on patients recovery; nurses demographic data. Journal of Nursing Standards. 2017;**9**:34

[29] Vera M. Appendectomy Nursing Care Plans. 2022. Available from: https://www.nursetogether.com/abdominal-pain-nursing-diagnosis-care-plan/

[30] Appendicitis. (n.d.). Johns Hopkins Medicine. Available from: https://www.hopkinsmedicine.org/health/conditions-and-diseases/appendicitis [Accessed December 3, 2022]

[31] Mayo Clinic. Appendicitis: Diagnosis and treatment. 2021. Available from: https://www.mayoclinic.org/diseases-conditions/appendicitis/diagnosis-treatment/drc-20369549 [Accessed: December 3, 2022]

[32] Sadia H, Kousar R, Azhar M, Waqas A, Gilani S. Assessment of nurses' knowledge and practices regarding prevention of surgical site infection. Saudi Journal of Medical Pharmaceutical Science. 2017;**36B**:585-595

[33] Davrieux C, Palermo M, Serra E, Houghton E, Acquafresca P, Finger C, et al. Stages and factors of the "Perioperative Process": Points in common with the aeronautical industry. Arquivos Brasileiros de Cirurgia Digestiva. 2019;**32**(1):e1423

[34] Bickley L, Szilagyi PG. Bates' Guide to Physical Examination and History-Taking. 12th ed. Philadelphia, PA: Wolters Kluwer; 2017

[35] Jarvis C. Physical Examination and Health Assessment. 6th ed. St. Louis: W.B. Saunders; 2012

[36] Doenges ME, Moorhouse MF, Murr AC. Nurse's Pocket Guide Diagnoses, Prioritized Interventions, and Rationales. 11th ed. F. A. Davis Company; 2008

[37] Partida JV. Appendicitis Management and Nursing Care Plan. 2018 NURSING PATH. Available from: https://www.nursingpath.in/2018/05/appendicitis-management-and-nursing.html [Accessed: December 3, 2022]

[38] Belleza M. Appendicitis. 2021. Available from: https://nurseslabs.com/appendicitis/ [Accessed: December 3, 2022]

[39] Sommers MS, Johnson SA, Beery TA. Diseases and Disorders a Nursing Therapeutics Manual. 3rd ed2008

[40] Allen E, Williams A, Jennings D, Stomski N, Goucke R, Toye C, et al. Revisiting the pain resource nurse role in sustaining evidence-based practice changes for pain assessment and management. Worldviews on Evidence-Based Nursing. 2018;**15**(5):368-376

[41] Famakinwa TT, Bello BG, Oyeniran YA, Okhiah O, Nwadike RN. Knowledge and practice of postoperative wound infection prevention among nurses in the surgical unit of a teaching hospital in Nigeria. International Journal of Basic, Applied Innovative Research. 2014;**3**(1):23-28

[42] Danwang C, Mazou TN, Tochie JN, et al. Global prevalence and incidence of surgical site infections after appendectomy: A systematic review and meta-analysis protocol. BMJ Open. 2018;**8**:e020101-e020e01. DOI: 10.1136/bmjopen-2017-020101

[43] Eta VEA, Namondo LA, Ngek ESN, Ngala E. Nurses' knowledge and practices on surgical site infections in Sub-Saharan Africa: The Case of Buea Regional Hospital, South West Region in Cameroon. American Journal of

Humanities and Social Sciences Research (AJHSSR). 2021;**6**:105-111

[44] Benson S, Powers J. Your Role in Infection Prevention: Nursing Made Incredible Easy. United State of America: Lippicontt Williams & Wilkins; 2011

[45] Harris CL, Kuhnke J, Haley J, Cross K, Somayaji R, Dubois J, et al. Best practice recommendations for the prevention and management of surgical wound complications. Canadian Association of Wound Care. 2018:1-66

[46] Famakinwa TT, Bello BG, Oyeniran YA, Okhiah O, Nwadike RN. Knowledge and practice of post-operative wound infection prevention among nurses in the surgical unit of a teaching hospital in Nigeria. International Journal of Basic, Applied and Innovation Research. 2014;**3**(1):23-28

[47] Diaz V, Newman J. Surgical site infection and prevention guidelines: A primer for certified registered nurse Anesthetists. AANA Journal. 2015;**83**:1